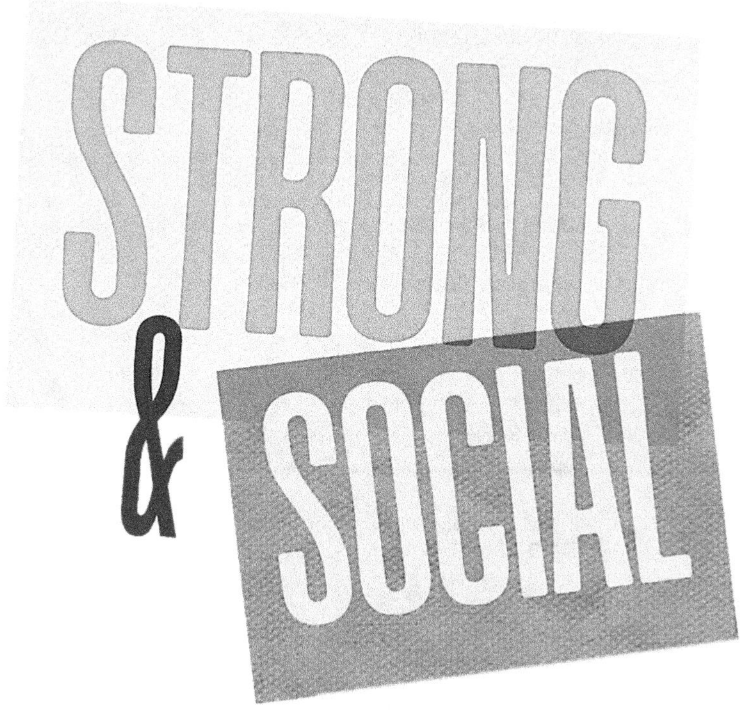

A GUIDE TO AGEING WELL THROUGH MOVEMENT AND SOCIAL CONNECTION

VAN MARINOS

FOREWORD BY ANDREW JOBLING

First Published in Australia in 2026
By Morpheus Publishing
Geelong Victoria 3216
www.morpheuspublishing.com.au

Paperback ISBN: 978-1-923650-20-6
Ebook: 978-1-923650-21-3
Ingram ISBN: 978-1-923650-22-0
Author: Van Marinos
Editor: Lynette Reurts
Cover Graphics: Mylan Carascal
Typesetting: Oseyi Okoeguale

A catalogue record for this book is available from the National Library of Australia.

DISCLAIMER

The information contained in this book is for general informational purposes only. The author and publisher are not offering any medical, legal or professional advice. While every effort has been made to ensure the accuracy and completeness of the information provided, the author and publisher assume no responsibility for errors or omissions or any outcomes or consequences resulting from using this book's content.

COPYRIGHT

DISTRIBUTION

This book is distributed by Morpheus Publishing and is available through authorised distributors, booksellers, Morpheus Publishing website.

COPYRIGHT PERMISSIONS

For copyright permissions or any other inquiries, please contact:

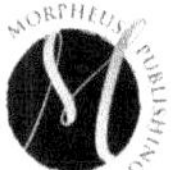

PUBLISHER: Morpheus Publishing
www.morpheuspublishing.com.au ||
hello@morpheuspublishing.com.au || +61403 564 942

AUTHOR: Van Marinos
https://www.morpheuspublishing.com.au/authors/van-marinos

CONTENTS

FOREWORD

Jim Rohn once said, *You become like the five people you spend the most time with.* More recently, James Clear stated, *You don't have to be the victim of your environment. You can also be the architect of it.* Both of these very credible authors, speakers, and thought-leaders have stated something that is universally true, no matter what you want for your life. That is, above everything else, the thing that will most determine the joy, fulfilment, wellbeing and outcomes in your life are the communities you join or develop.

It took many years for me to work this out as I pushed, struggled, crawled, and aspired to be successful in life, thinking I had to do it all on my own. I was wrong. If only I knew then what Van so wonderfully describes in this book, my journey would have been more fun and fulfilling and who knows how things may have turned out. Maybe I would have been more successful in my professional sporting career. Potentially, I would have had a better business experience. I would definitely have made less mistakes, and had more support on my journey. Today, as an author, speaker, mentor, podcaster, and someone who has been in the health and wellbeing industry for many decades, I understand the power of community.

The reality is that knowledge alone is not the answer. We know everything we need to know, or can access that information at any time, to get any results we want in life. That being the case, why are so many people struggling with their health, their relationships, their finances, and in many other areas of life? As a personal trainer, speaker and author, every day I teach people, in some forum, how they can be fitter, healthier, happier, and more abundant in life. Why do so few actually apply the information consistently? The answer is community.

When I met Van Marinos, I was immediately inspired and impressed. We connected on LinkedIn and our first conversation got my mind racing. As he spoke about his passion, his family, and his business *Community Moves,* I knew this was a man I wanted in my community. He explained many things to me that he touches on in this book, about the evolution of his business and how it grew so organically to multiple studios today and is still growing. His mission: to give people in the more mature stage of life the opportunity to live with health, energy, and wellbeing for many years and defy the loss of function and quality of life that comes to many people with age.

When he explained to me his business development and onboarding strategy, I was inspired. He had created a place where people came, not only for fitness, strength, and wellbeing, but more so for the feeling of belonging to the fun, caring, and inclusive community. The community is so together, and the loyalty for Van and his team so strong, that it is mainly clients and people within the existing community who refer *Community Moves* to others, and even take them through the onboarding process when they join. Now that is a community where people feel valued. The clients arrange the social events and set the mood and tone for the business, and the result has been rapid growth and incredible success. I immediately invited Van to be a guest on my podcast, and we then started discussing how I could support him in writing a book. That conversation was at the end of 2024, and that book you are reading today, published in early 2026.

As I helped him write this book, I read it and loved it. Yes, it is an awesome book about fitness, strength, mobility, flexibility, balance, longevity, and physical wellbeing. But it is so much more! It is about connection, inspiration, gratitude, and building strong communities. The more I learn, the longer I live, and the more I see, the more I know that these are the things most consistent with living a life of joyful longevity. In other words, you can eat the right foods and do the right exercise, but if you lack connection, community, and gratitude, you will struggle.

You may have heard of 'Blue Zones'. From www.longevity.direct:

> *In certain pockets of the world, people routinely live past 100 in remarkable health. These areas, dubbed 'Blue Zones' by researcher Dan Buettner, share fascinating commonalities – particularly in how their communities function. From Okinawa, Japan to Sardinia, Italy, these longevity hotspots prove that living longer isn't just about diet or exercise – it's about the power of human connection.*

Strong and Social, by Van Marinos, will inspire you, inform you, and empower you to start living a life and developing a 'blue zone' in your own home and community. Read these pages with anticipation that it will help you, your family and your community, and create a powerful ripple effect that will impact millions of lives all around the world.

Andrew Jobling
www.andrewjobling.com.au

SECTION 1

CONTEXT AND FRAMEWORK

INTRODUCTION

There was a brief period when I thought I might be able to save him. In April of 2024, my father, aged 75, was diagnosed with stage 4 lung cancer — it was terminal.

As an exercise scientist with a couple of tertiary qualifications, decades of experience in the health and fitness industry, and a solid understanding of the research and science surrounding chronic disease, I should have known that this was essentially a death sentence, and that the 6 to 12-month timeline was exactly what we could expect.

Perhaps it was naivety, arrogance, ignorance, or just pure blind hope, but I was determined to get him at least a few more years. I thought I could beat the statistics and perform some sort of exercise-powered miracle that would keep my dad with us, and the cancer at bay.

I failed. He died at home, surrounded by family, smothered in love, at a moment of his choosing, on September 13th, just 6 months after his diagnosis.

At this point, you could be forgiven for thinking, 'What's this got to do with exercise and social interaction!?' Well… a few things.

Dad (and Mum) were a large part of the reason I ended up building my health and fitness business, Community Moves, that caters specifically to older adults. They were representative of the majority of older Australians who had never really done much structured exercise, had a number of chronic health issues, and didn't really know where to go or what to do about it.

Once they'd begun exercising regularly, it was the strength of the community and the social connections (as well as the pressure from their son) that kept them coming consistently. And, despite Dad's final 6 months of life, the 6 years prior, where he had been regularly exercising with a group of his peers, represented a period where he felt the fittest, healthiest, and happiest he had in a long time. He became part of our wonderful gym community.

It was this very community that wrapped their arms around my mother and I when he passed, and the one that continues to support us through our grief, as they do with each other through all manner of life's barbs and betrayals.

This is the real story.

Yes, the exercise stuff is hugely important, as we'll cover in the coming chapters, but it is the social and community aspects of Community Moves that I've witnessed that drove me to write this book and share my experience with you.

It's the stories of support, friendship, and even companionship that have formed on the gym floor and expanded well beyond our walls.

It's the story of how these relationships and the community that binds them feed back into the exercise program, and result in health behaviour changes that many would admit they never expected.

For us, the integration of group exercise and social interaction for older adults has proven to be a winning recipe, and like all recipes, it has the potential to be replicated to achieve similar results. We'll look at each of these ingredients in isolation, and in detail, and then dive into the reasons that combining them is like combining custard and jelly, or turkey and cranberry sauce, or… (enter favourite combination here). It just works.

In planning this book, I asked a number of Community Moves members to write about their experiences with us to provide some real-world examples of how powerful the combination of exercise and social connection can be. This is not, by any means, meant to come across as a set of testimonials or a promotion of Community Moves. I simply felt it would be the best way to tell the story.

I was tempted to edit their contributions and develop a narrative for each one, creating a section at the end of each with key messages and takeaways. I decided against it, opting to leave their stories exactly as they were given to me. I'll leave it to you to find the messages within.

Before we get to that, I'd like to share a little bit about myself and my journey to this point. I'm not a writer or public figure with a distinguished career or compelling story that people necessarily want to hear. I'm simply an exercise professional with a passion for helping people improve the way they age. I don't have knowledge of a special fitness secret that isn't already out there, and don't have as many letters after my name as many others.

I'm writing this book because I have an important message and story to share and want to contribute something positive to the world.

Growing up, I was always into sports and physical activity. Mum represented Australia in synchronised swimming, and Dad was a sports nut. I fell in love with football (soccer) at a young age and wanted to play professionally when I got older.

By the time I was in my late teens, it was clear that I wasn't going to make it to the elite level. I was a good player, but a late developer physically. This led to a lack of confidence, which ultimately resulted in me dropping out of representative football and letting the dream go with it.

However, this lack of confidence and perceived physical inadequacy led me to pursue other activities, namely strength and conditioning training.

It was pretty much love at first workout.

By the time I was in my 20s, I was studying Human Movement and Health Education at Sydney University, working in a gym, coaching junior football teams, and captaining a local league football club. Recognised for my physical presence and combative nature, it was a stark contrast to the little, baby-faced teen that hid on the field ten years beforehand.

My love and passion for football eventually landed me a role with Football Federation Australia (FFA). A dream come true. I'd spent 7 years in teaching, coach education, and junior sport development, and even completed a master's degree in Sports Coaching with Griffith University, before finally landing the role as FFA's National MiniRoos Manager.

Throughout this period, I'd still managed to keep my health and fitness hat on, running my own personal training business and teaching group exercise classes.

As National MiniRoos Manager, I helped build our current national junior football program and am extremely proud of the work I did there. But, as with most jobs in sport, the higher you go, the more likely it is that you have to swap your football boots for business shoes (unless, of course, you are a career coach).

So, after a decade in sports development and coach education, it was time for a new challenge.

I knew that I wanted to run my own business, and knew that I wanted it to be back in health and fitness. I also knew that I wanted to do something that was aligned with my values and skill set. I was never motivated by money, hated the Instagram model, self-loving side of the fitness industry, didn't want to work in elite sport, and wanted to put some good into the world.

The Australian fitness industry trends and national health statistics all pointed to a need for more health and fitness services catered to older Australians.

Dad had survived a heart attack in his 50s and had Leukaemia; he'd changed his lifestyle a bit but was doing little to improve his health. He wasn't interested in going to a regular gym, it just wasn't his scene. Mum walked the dog regularly and attended occasional gym classes, where she'd inevitably end up hurting her back whilst trying to keep up with the other 50 participants in the room. She also ended up with osteoporosis.

They were my avatars, as well as my biggest supporters.

I went back to personal training full time, which allowed me to do some experiential research, train my body to get up at 4:30am every day again, up-skill in all the right areas, and build a business plan. In 2017, I ran a pilot program for local over-50s, which validated my business and market assumptions, and in 2018, Community Moves Health & Fitness was born.

Community Moves Health & Fitness was all about providing an environment and exercise program specifically built to serve the local over-50s.

The sessions incorporated all aspects of fitness and movement, catered to all abilities and fitness levels, and addressed some of the most common musculoskeletal issues experienced by older adults.

Over the next year or so, the business grew pretty steadily. Many of our members shared similar frustrations about the lack of appropriate programs like this in mainstream gyms. Many had been injured in the past or had bad fitness experiences and were reluctant to return to exercise in an environment that they didn't feel comfortable in. And all of our members began improving not only their physical fitness but their mental health as well.

We held regular health workshops on topics like breathing, posture, and nutrition (this one drew the biggest crowd). It was now clear that most of our members, and many other local community members who attended our events, were hungry for more information and services that would help them stay healthier for longer.

One thing that I had only paid a small amount of attention to while planning was the 'community and social' side of the business. In my experience, which in hindsight had no relevance to my customers, gym members didn't really socialise that much and weren't necessarily looking for that experience as part of their membership.

So, I was initially a little surprised, and extremely pleased, at the positive impact that the program was having on our members' social and emotional health. New friendship groups were being formed, strong connections were being established, and a beautiful 'community' of like-minded local over-50s was being built.

Then… a viral outbreak at a food market in Wuhan, China, changed the world.

The gym was closed for three months, and I feared the worst. We weren't set up to deliver our services online; after all, online fitness programs were only for young people, right? WRONG!

Within a week of being closed, we'd built an online portal for our members where we uploaded three, one hour-long sessions each week that could be completed from the comfort of their living room. We also ran three live sessions each week via Zoom to try and keep some form of social connection and solidarity. We partnered with a local gym equipment store and organised a discounted exercise equipment pack for Community Moves members.

Over the twelve-week lockdown, we had about an 85% participation rate in our online programs in one form or another. Despite a few technical speed bumps, the experience was fantastic and further fortified my understanding of the strength of community and the importance of social connection.

Fast forward to today, and we've got three studios in Sydney's north, all helping local over 50s improve their physical, mental, and social health. We host regular social events like trivia nights, barefoot bowls, dance and dine… the list goes on. Our members run a number of intra clubs, including book clubs, foodie groups, and movie clubs. They actively engage in local charity drives, get together for lunches, have coffee together after class, and share their lives over numerous WhatsApp group chats. They support one another when one of them is sick and deliver groceries to each other if they are unable to shop for themselves.

All the while, they see each other three times a week at the gym for their regular dose of exercise.

That is where the magic lies, and what this book is about: the powerful combination of exercise and community, and the personal stories of some of those who have benefited from it.

It wasn't enough to save my dad from dying, but it certainly added life, vitality, and quality to his final years. It enabled him to keep chasing his grandkids and spend time with his family unencumbered by physical limitation, to continue to work on passion projects that required a certain level of mobility and fitness, and to attend various social events that he never would have before; and, I think, it brought him and mum a little closer together.

If you'd have asked him what he would have wanted from his final years, I'm pretty sure his list wouldn't have been too different from that.

Hopefully, when you think about what you want to do in your final years, you also think about the physical, social, and community health requirements that will support your goals.

If work needs to be done to bring your goals and health requirements closer together, this book is for you.

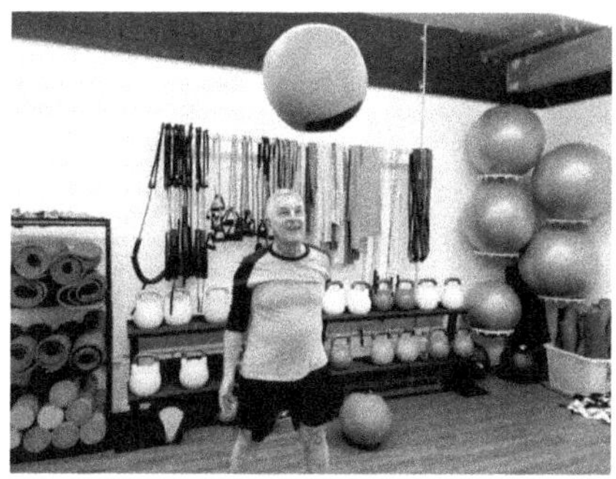

Dad enjoying himself during an exercise session at the original studio, who'd have ever thought!

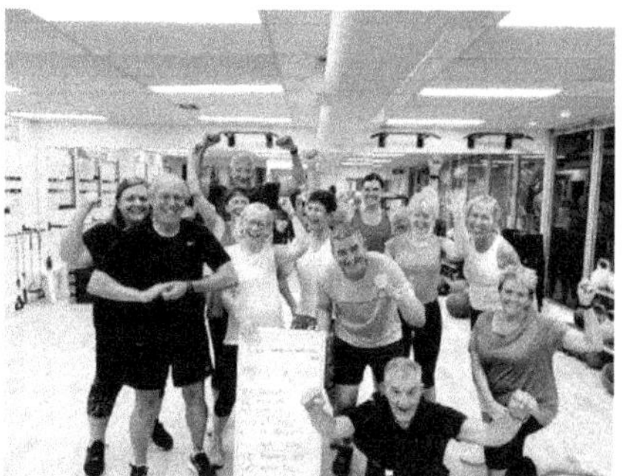

Taken after one of our more intense sessions. Dad loved keeping up with this group.

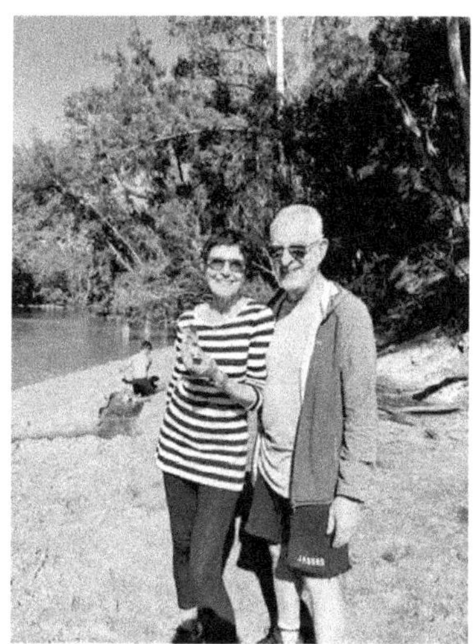

Mum and Dad at Colo River, camping with the family shortly after his first round of chemo.

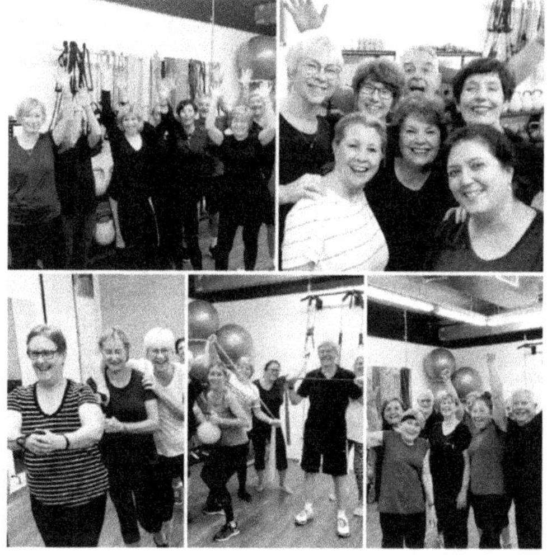

Early days at Community Moves. Many of these members still come to the gym and are now dear friends of my mother's...and mine.

CHAPTER 1

GREATEST TIME TO BE ALIVE... IS IT?

Just over 100 years ago, our average life expectancy was between 30 and 40 years. In 2026, Australians can now expect to live to somewhere between 80 to 85 years[1].

Modern science, advances in medicine, better education, effective sanitation, and improved living standards have enabled us to increase our life expectancy at a fairly steady rate over the last few decades.

At this point, I feel it necessary to highlight that these figures are not representative of our whole population, especially our indigenous peoples. Their life expectancy is, to our shame, far lower than that of most Australians. This story may be well beyond the scope of this book, but it will never be far from the mind of the author.

Always Was, Always Will Be, Aboriginal Land

Despite the differences in the life expectancies of different demographics, the fact remains that we are living longer. However, this doesn't necessarily mean that we are living better. An increase in the length of our lives does not always equate to an increase in the quality of our lives. Older adults in Australia have some of the worst health statistics of the whole population and are more likely to suffer from one or more chronic lifestyle diseases.

At the same time that the steady march of science and technology has driven improvements in healthcare and living standards of much of the Western world, it has also heavily influenced the way we live, work, move, eat, connect, and survive. And not necessarily for the better.

In his book, Death by Comfort, Paul Taylor does a great job of detailing the impact that our more sedentary lives are having on our physical health and function. In modern society, it is not uncommon for someone to sit in the car on the way to work, sit at their desk all day, sit in the car again on the way home, sit for dinner, and sit on the couch and watch TV before going to bed.

This level of inactivity was certainly not what the body was designed for and can result in a range of health issues. As Taylor likes to remind us, the human genome requires us to be highly physically active for normal functioning, and our current lifestyles are massively betraying this pact.

Many of these issues may not be so noticeable in our younger years, but after years of poor physical habits, the body you retire with will tell the story of how it was treated throughout its preceding years.

Starting your retirement, or having to continue working, with a body that is falling apart and is a constant source of pain and discomfort, is surely not going to make a positive contribution to those 'twilight' years. Not to mention the impact it can have on your bank account. According to the Australian Institute of Health and Welfare, in the 2022-23 period, Australia's total health expenditure averaged $9,597 per person.

Technology and science (and capitalism) have also dramatically changed the way we eat. Highly processed foods with little nutritional value have been mass-produced and marketed very effectively. Similarly, Australia is now facing a severe overweight and obesity epidemic and a rise in chronic conditions such as Type II Diabetes and Metabolic Syndrome that are linked to poor nutritional and physical activity habits.

Conversely, improved nutrition and dietary practices are directly linked to better health outcomes and reductions in risks for some cancers, cardiovascular disease, diabetes, and other chronic diseases.

However, despite this knowledge and having greater access to a wide range of fresh produce and groceries than ever, older adults in Australia exhibit the poorest nutritional habits of all population segments [2].

Potential reasons for this could range from a lack of nutrition education or reduced appetite due to changed physical activity patterns, to the practical limitations associated with diet and dental health. Budgetary concerns also factor in here as fresh produce is often more expensive than less nutritious alternatives.

Social isolation and loneliness, and the associated decline in mental health, have long been areas of concern for older adults. Higher likelihood of divorce or becoming widowed, empty nesting, diminishing friendship networks, retirement… The list of causes goes on.

Then, 2020 hit us with Covid-19, forcing everyone into lockdown.

Being unable to see friends and family, or even attend a single weekly event with some social interaction, would test the resolve and mental fortitude of a Navy SEAL, let alone that of someone who was already considered at risk. Throw the challenge of learning and adapting to new technologies into the mix, and we start to paint a pretty unhappy picture.

So, although we are living longer, the likelihood that we are unfit, unhealthy, and unhappy is much higher in our later years than it is when we are younger.

This doesn't have to be the case, however.

Yes, everyone is going to die, and everyone is going to get old. Humankind has been searching unsuccessfully for the elixir of life since the dawn of time. However, how we choose to die, or more appropriately, how we choose to live, can have a massive impact on our quality of life as we age.

Our body and our brain are amazing structures. They are capable of adapting, growing, modifying, and responding to various stimuli at all ages.

This book is about helping as many people as possible face the second half of their life armed with some powerful tools to keep them running at their best and thriving well beyond their twilight years. We might not all get there, but what a fun game to play!

My hope and vision are that by helping to improve the health and lives of as many individuals as possible, we are able to improve the health of our communities, and as a result, start to make a significant impact on the alarming health statistics of our older Australians.

CHAPTER 2

CATHERINE

Catherine has been a member at Community Moves for over 6 years. Like many of our former nurses, and most of our members for that matter, she has a kind heart and generous spirit. Her story is likely representative of many older adults but exemplifies the value in finding new connections later in life. This is her story.

In 1964, I decided to fulfil my desire to become a Nurse. I contacted the Mater Misericordiae Hospital and placed my name on the Waiting List. In October that year, I was accepted, and that was the beginning of a wonderful career.

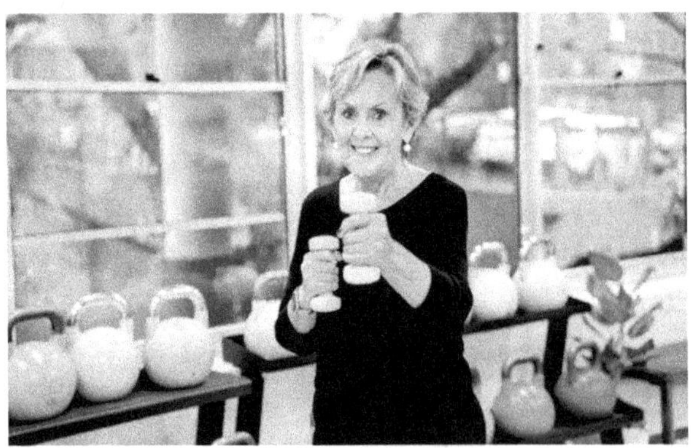

Catherine striking a pose at our Neutral Bay studio.

I completed my General Nursing, which took four amazing years to complete. So next was Midwifery, a further year of study at St Margaret's Hospital, completing that in 1969, then over to the Paediatric Unit to study in the Neonatal Unit. Completing that, I was then asked to stay on in the Maternity Hospital to set up an Acute Care area.

I got married in late 1970, and due to now living in Wollstonecraft and expecting our first precious baby, I returned to the Mater, which was close to home. The next years were extremely busy as we moved from state to state with my husband's career, and now having four children and working in hospitals in many states. There was not a lot of ME time, but I did play tennis as often as possible. Walking whenever I could was my sanity.

After many years with knee problems, I was advised in 2016 to have Bilateral Knee Replacements, not an easy decision, but necessary.

In 2018, I decided to finally change to part-time work at the Mater Hospital. Wondering what to do in my retirement, I was walking through Neutral Bay Shops and saw a group exercising in a room in The Grove. I decided that it looked like a great group of women, and so I made one of the best decisions of my life. Joining Community Moves Gym has not only helped me get over two pretty big surgeries but also has continued to encourage me to stay physically fit.

I was lucky to be diagnosed with early-stage Lung Cancer in 2023 and had a Lobe of my Lung removed. I don't think I would have recovered so well had I not been attending regular exercise classes.

Retiring from work is not easy, as those people you worked with will always be special, but the contacts do lessen as we take a different road.

From that first visit to the gym, I was incredibly lucky to meet some wonderful, amazing women. I have continued to develop an incredible social network, which I treasure. We are there to support each other in good times, but also in difficult times. We enjoy walks, dinners, theatre visits and many more adventures.

Many do voluntary and community work, helping in many special ways. I have been fortunate to visit weekly a beautiful friend who, sadly, developed Dementia. We met at Community Moves, and our relationship has been strong ever since. My beautiful dog Tilly and I go to the home she lives in, take her for a good hour or so walk, and then we have coffee. We then let the other residents have some cuddles with Tilly.

CHAPTER 3

AGEING UNGRACEFULLY

In 1966, the University of Texas Southwestern Medical School conducted an experiment on five 20-year-old men to examine the effects of bed rest and endurance training on their cardiorespiratory fitness. They then followed up with the same men some 30 years later to examine the effects of ageing on the same system [3][4].

The findings were astonishing and had an immediate and lasting clinical impact, helping to reduce sedentary time in the management of acute and chronic medical conditions.

Get this…. three weeks of bed rest did more damage to the cardiorespiratory system than 30 years of ageing. Let that sink in for a moment.

Twenty one days of doing nothing was worse for our cardiorespiratory fitness than 10,950 days of normal ageing.

It is also worth noting that after the three-week bed rest, they embarked on an eight-week endurance training program and all experienced improvements in their cardiorespiratory fitness beyond baseline.

However, that's not the point. The point is that being highly sedentary can have hugely detrimental effects on our health. There are similar studies that highlight the effect of bed rest and low physical activity rates on muscle mass, strength, balance… the list goes on. Nothing good comes from being physically inactive.

A common conversation I have with members of Community Moves, who have recently returned from a lazy holiday or medical event requiring absence from the gym and abstinence from exercise, is about how noticeably deconditioned they feel. It is quite a shocking revelation when you realise how hard fitness can be to gain and maintain, but how easy it is to lose.

With the rise of technology, namely screens and similar devices, has come the fall in physical activity rates. Most people spend their working days sitting in front of a computer screen, and many don't even need to leave their homes to do it. Children can spend hours on end playing video games from the comfort of their couch without interacting with anyone. We can order food to our door and outsource almost any service we need to someone else.

I recently drove past a bus stop outside a high school, and every single teenager was standing or sitting against a wall, with their heads drooped over their phone screens. I remember playing soccer and chasing my mates when I was waiting for the bus after school. Our behaviours have been insidiously changed by technology.

We are also inherently lazy. In evolutionary terms, we were made to grow, hunt, gather, survive, and procreate. Resources were sparse, so wasting time and energy doing anything else was pointless.

In modern-day society, particularly in Western cultures, we have all the food we need at the push of a button and all the comfort of a climate-controlled space wherever we go. The perfect combination for our 'lazy' genome to bask in.

So, what's the problem?

Well, although our ancestors, the 'hunter-gatherers', spent a lot of time resting and conserving energy when and where needed, they also spent a heck of a lot more time being physically active.

One of the last 'hunter-gatherer' tribes in existence today is the Hadza people of Tanzania. Whenever someone writes about the difference between our current activity rates and those of our ancestors, they will inevitably reference this group of people and the research findings that several studies into their lifestyle have collected.

Amongst the various contrasts in lifestyle, such as diet and social cohesion, is the stark contrast in physical activity rates. According to Pontzer et al.'s [5] research on the Hadza's activity patterns, the men averaged approximately 13,000–15,000 steps/day, and women averaged approximately 10,000–12,000 steps/day.

Of their daily activity, approximately 60-90 minutes was spent at vigorous intensity effort and 240-280 minutes was spent at moderate intensity.

According to the research, the Hadza have low instances of cardiovascular disease, diabetes, and hypertension and remain active into old age.

In comparison, the average adult in western societies averages 4000-6000 steps/day, if they're lucky. Australia's Physical Activity recommendations for adults are 150 minutes of moderate activity or 75 minutes of vigorous activity a week. Yes, that's a week! And only around 25% of us are meeting those guidelines [6][7].

According to the Australian Bureau of Statistics (ABS), in 2022, almost all individuals aged 65 years and over (99.2%) reported having at least one long-term health condition[8].

These conditions often include chronic diseases such as arthritis, cardiovascular disease, diabetes, and respiratory disorders.

This means that for the majority of older Australians, by the time they reach retirement age, they will already suffer from one or more chronic conditions. What's even more concerning is that many of those whom I speak to consider it a normal part of ageing. It's as though we just accept that after a certain age, our bodies are going to pack it in, and we'll have to negotiate the final decades of our lives managing these conditions as best we can.

This is not normal. All that's really happening is our bodies are finally showing symptoms of the damage we've been doing to them for the previous 40-50 years.

Now, before you get your knickers in a knot, I'm not suggesting that if we exercised all our lives, we'd never get sick or suffer from any chronic conditions. There are so many factors that influence our health — diet, stress, genetics, just to name a few. However, surely, we can do better as a society to help improve the poor statistics around physical activity and chronic disease prevalence in older adults.

Australia currently spends just 2% of its health budget on prevention, far below other nations like the UK (4%) and Canada (nearly 6%). In other words: for every dollar we spend keeping people healthy, we spend fifty dollars treating diseases that have already developed.

Take osteoarthritis as an example. In 2020–21, we spent $4.3 billion managing this condition — almost 3% of the entire health budget, and nearly a third of all musculoskeletal expenditure. That's an extraordinary cost for a condition where early movement, strength, and lifestyle interventions can dramatically change long-term outcomes.

The Australian Institute of Health and Welfare reported that in 2022–2023, the average healthcare spend per capita was approximately $9500. Considering that older adults are likely to spend more on health care than younger people, I think it would be fair to assume that this number would be significantly higher for older Australians.

I think it would also be fair to assume that most older adults are not spending close to $9500 per year on preventative health measures.

Just as a bit of a thought experiment… Using those same numbers, say 3% of Australia's health budget ($4.3 billion in 2020–21) was allocated to increasing older Australians' physical activity rates rather than treatment options for Osteoarthritis (OA). Divided among approximately 4.3 million older Australians, each individual would be allocated $1,000.

I know there are a lot of variables and holes in this statement, and it's not very fair on those suffering from OA, but just continue to indulge me for a moment.

Research has consistently proven that regular physical activity significantly reduces the risk of developing and managing almost all chronic lifestyle diseases. Imagine if that $4.3 billion was spent on subsidising gym memberships or helping provide greater access to physical activity opportunities for older adults.

If we wanted to be really Draconian, we could go a step further and look at linking the funding to tax incentives or pension allocations. "Gym Goer? Get Your Taxes Lower." or "Three to five gym sessions a week? A higher pension you shall reap!"

Clearly, I'm not in marketing or public policy. But you get the drift.

Corny tag lines aside, imagine if we could increase the number of older adults who meet the recommended physical activity guidelines from 25% to 50%. The implications this would have for the health system would be huge. Not only would there be less spending on health treatment for each individual, but there would be a ripple effect that is hard to quantify. Greater health outcomes mean longer time in the workforce and increased productivity, more time travelling and chasing grandkids, more time actively contributing to local communities, greater mental health outcomes, increased opportunities for intergenerational connection and collaboration… the advantages are endless, and we all stand to benefit.

Unfortunately, it's just not that simple. Health behaviour change is hard, really hard. We'll look at some models of health behaviour change in more detail later but expecting individuals to fight against their evolutionary biases, change their sedentary-based lifestyles, and lean into the discomfort of regular physical activity because they may reduce their risk of early death and improve their quality of life is unrealistic and obviously hasn't worked. Especially when talking about the segment of the population that has been building poor health habits for the longest period of time.

It's not an education problem. Everyone knows they need to do more exercise. Just like we know, we need to eat healthier foods, sit less, move more, drink less alcohol, quit smoking, snack on fewer treats… blah, blah, blah.

The problem is that exercise is a stress.

It's a hormetic stress, which means that when delivered in small doses, it produces a response in the body that is actually beneficial. And like many other hormetic stressors, there is generally a dose response. The more difficult it is and the greater the level of exposure (to a point), the greater the adaptive response.

However, it is a stress nonetheless. The majority of people, not only older adults, but toddlers through to centenarians, will generally avoid this kind of stress like the plague. Exercise stress is uncomfortable, it's difficult, it often hurts, you get sweaty, you make weird noises, you often have to wear tight clothes, and you have to do it multiple times a week… forever!

No wonder people don't want to do it.

There are some people, myself included, who actually enjoy it. We are definitely in the minority but we do exist. Most of us end up, like me, working in the health and fitness industry, trying to drag the nonbelievers with us. It's a hard sell and getting harder. The pharmaceutical industry is constantly producing drugs that attempt to mimic some of the benefits of exercise and put them in the shape of a pill, new technologies are forever emerging claiming to provide the greatest results for the least amount of effort, and I'm quite certain that AI will soon be able to do the exercise for us, just like it is doing for so much else.

For now, though, there is nothing out there that comes close to matching the real thing. The trick is to find a way to make exercise more palatable and more enjoyable so that we get the right amount of stress, but without the overwhelming feelings of discomfort.

This is where I believe, particularly for a lot of older adults, the role of social connection and community building becomes hugely important. Finding people to exercise with who are at the same stage of life, share similar interests (and often socio-economic status), and are from the same geographical area can make it all seem a little less stressful. In fact, as I'll go on to show you, it can actually be one of the most powerful tools when it comes to health behaviour change, specifically exercise adherence.

Yes, as a society, we are ageing ungracefully. We are generally unfit, unhealthy, and socially disconnected. The beautiful thing is, though, we are one of the most adaptive species on the planet. Our bodies will try to adapt to pretty much whatever we throw at them, at any stage of life. We'll do a bit of a deep dive into the power of social connection and community a little later, but for the next few chapters, we'll look at the incredible benefits of exercise and what you can do to start moving the needle in the right direction.

CHAPTER 4

JOHN

Comparing the John that walked through our doors many years ago to the man he is now is like comparing chalk and cheese. As you'll read, his story is typical of many older adults who have spent a lifetime prioritising their career ahead of their health. Stress, weight gain, physical inactivity and poor nutritional habits all caught up with him.

Fortunately, he is a determined and disciplined man, with a wonderfully supportive and caring wife. He turned things around and is now lean, fit, and strong. When he started with Community Moves, he had a double chin; now, he does chin-ups.

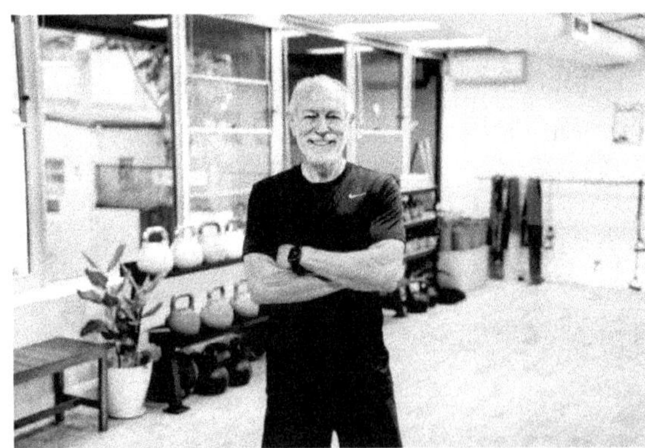

John standing proud at Community Moves Neutral Bay

As a youngster growing up in Western Australia, I was a sports fanatic, actively involved in athletics until my mid-teens and Aussie rules football until my early twenties. As such, I followed a very disciplined exercise regime until the end of my Aussie rules pursuits – then, unfortunately, submitting to a more sedentary and less healthy lifestyle.

During my twenties, I started to focus on a career in Financial Services, and then life became even more serious with marriage and the arrival of our first child.

While my career in Financial Services blossomed, it was at the expense of my health. Long hours, lots of travel both interstate and international, dinners and alcohol, stress, and plenty of excuses because there was no time for exercise or a healthy diet.

Over the years, I did try on occasion to introduce exercise into my weekly regimen, but like many fad diets, this only lasted for relatively short periods of time. As a result, I gained quite a bit of weight, and while I knew what I needed to do, it was easier in my mind to just block it out and concentrate on work.

I have always been fortunate not to suffer any serious joint issues, however, my unhealthy lifestyle more than likely led to several other ailments. Heart issues and a pacemaker at the age of 49, prostate problems, inflammatory issues and sepsis, all culminating in retiring from full-time work in January 2016 at the age of 62.

The year following my retirement, Jane and I spent quite a bit of time travelling, and at about the same time, I started to think more about exercise. No work excuses now, but in reality, the exercise was just some walking and regular golf — nothing too physical, and of course, little attention to a healthy diet and unfortunately, still overweight.

At this stage, we had just started to think about downsizing and a potential move to the lower North Shore. There was really nothing holding us back; the kids had left home, and we really did not have a circle of friends in the area. Socially, our friends in Sydney were people we had met through the kids' school days or ex-work colleagues. We had left our closest network of friends when we moved from Perth in 1994, and while we never felt lonely, the friendships we had in Sydney were just not the same as those in Perth. In many respects, this made family even more important, and of course, our kids had now 'flown the coop', so we were somewhat on our own, so to speak!

Community Moves came into our lives about five years ago. Jane had been going to Vision in Lindfield prior to us moving to Neutral Bay, and following a recommendation, she decided to try it out. A couple of months in, Jane suggested that I give CM a go and in typical macho fashion, I dismissed the idea. I'm not sure why — maybe Jane's persistence and her knowing better than I what would be good for me — but eventually I decided to give it a go. So off I go, still overweight and not following a healthy diet — and surprise, surprise, I start to enjoy this place.

While still not doing much about diet, I am now doing regular exercise, and once again to my surprise, meeting some very nice, like-minded people.

But alas, all's not well, and within a relatively short time of joining CM, my health deteriorates. I'm getting awful pains in the chest, and on 23 December 2020, I ended up in the hospital — the unhealthy lifestyle has finally caught up with me. Within a period of 8 months, I had my first stent, then another two, and ultimately cardiac bypass surgery – a bit of a wake-up call if I ever needed one, and the recovery was painful.

Following a period of recovery, I'm now determined to change things. First thing is to give up alcohol — yes, go cold turkey — I just can't trust myself to do it any other way, and 4 years on, I still don't touch alcohol. Turns out that's not as big a deal as I thought it would be, and while I don't begrudge anyone choosing to drink, it's fantastic waking up every morning with a clear head and not feeling sluggish.

A healthier diet was the next challenge! The cardiac rehab dietitians told me all the things that I already knew but had failed to adhere to in the past. Diet remains my biggest challenge in leading a healthy lifestyle, but CM, through the Nutrition & Accountability program, has helped immensely, not so much in knowing what not to eat (hey, we all know that stuff), but more about portion sizes, healthy snacks, etc. And the daily check-ins, someone to keep me honest!

As for exercise, the CM program is perfect for me — the blend of regular sessions, CM Plus, Advanced Strength, and Pilates (Pilates — did I say that? Who would have ever thought!) is, in my opinion, a great mix of exercises for this age demographic. The strange thing is, I now look forward to going to exercise classes, whereas once I was always looking for an easy out.

Apart from the benefits of exercise, I have wondered at times why I enjoy going to CM and I conclude that the answer is obvious. It really is about the people, the banter, the friendships, and the coffee after classes. The feeling of being part of something bigger — an extended family, if you like. A family that is caring, giving and looks out for each other

Socially, we feel that our lives are full. We now have a group of very dear friends with whom we catch up regularly, travel with and share many laughs.

CM should have come into my life many years earlier — or maybe I just should have paid more attention to these things earlier on in life. Certainly, downsizing to Neutral Bay and discovering CM has had a profound impact on our lives.

CHAPTER 5

EXERCISE: THE MAGIC PILL

Dr Kenneth Cooper, affectionately known as the godfather of aerobics, is credited with coining the saying, "You don't stop exercising because you grow old, you grow old because you stop exercising."

I have no idea who he was referring to when he said it or how he meant it to be interpreted, but I love it. It's simple, accurate, and stands the test of time. What I do know for certain is that humans are built to move. In fact, we evolved over millions of years to function optimally whilst being highly physically active.

Our brains grew bigger and bigger, fuelled by our increased movement capacity. We transitioned from predominately moving around on all fours to standing and moving on two legs. We developed a huge capacity for walking and running long distance, strong muscles for sprinting short distances and carrying heavy things, and a combination of joints, bones, and muscles that are organised in such a way that we are/were capable of moving in the most extraordinary ways whilst completing the most amazing feats of physical performance. And that's just scratching the surface.

All these physical characteristics are supported by thousands of cellular interactions and processes that enable our body and brain to communicate, decide a course of action, act, review, adapt, and return to baseline without any conscious control.

Let's take the familiar fight-or-flight response as an example. When a threat is perceived, adrenaline and cortisol are released into the bloodstream, leading to an increase in blood glucose levels. This provides a rapid source of energy, enabling us to react quickly with speed, power, and urgency — all within seconds. Once the threat subsides, hormone levels return to baseline, and excess glucose is either utilised for immediate energy or stored in the liver and muscles as glycogen. All without us really doing anything.

All of these evolutionary traits and capabilities were developed over a very long period of time and are expected to be used regularly. They are not optional extras, and they all work together in beautiful harmony.

For the human genome, exercise and physical activity are not just optional; they are essential. There is not one single physiological system that remains unaffected by exercise.

So, unless you are going to live like the Hadza people and get enough varied physical activity to nourish the body whilst completing activities of daily living, structured exercise and planned physical activity are the next best thing.

For the purpose of this book, we'll look at just a few of the key areas of physical fitness that need to be addressed, why these are so important for older adults, and some practical applications. Although I have ordered these by level of importance from my perspective, they are all critical and a case could probably be made for each to be at the top of the list.

1) Strength & Muscle Building
2) Cardiorespiratory Fitness
3) Stability & Balance

4) Mobility & Flexibility

Each of these categories could be the sole topic of entire books in their own right. There is no limit to the amount of detail, science, and practical applications that could be covered on each topic, but I've chosen to keep it fairly basic.

Hopefully, this book will encourage you to seek out more information and work with people who can help you put it into practice.

In saying that, there is a full chapter dedicated to strength and muscle mass coming up. I have double-clicked on this area of physical fitness as it is, in my opinion, the one that older adults tend to need the most, and the one that confers the greatest health benefits.

At the end of Section 2, you'll find some simple tests you can perform to assess your level of function across these areas, including your breathing.

PETER

This is just a short message I received from one of our members that I wanted to include, as Peter's journey is such a common one. His body had started to let him down, and he was faced with a serious health condition. He realised he needed to do more to improve his health, and found somewhere he could exercise that supported his goals. He now views his exercise regime as part of his lifestyle in helping him to keep doing the things he loves outside of the gym.

In early 2023, I suffered an illness which led to me ceasing my part-time work for nearly nine months and also giving up my weekly swimming activity.

Towards the end of that year, I became fully recovered medically, but the long period of physical inactivity had taken its toll, although at the time I didn't recognise it.

I had started swimming again and partly returned to work, but I was not really at the same level of physical capability and mental wellbeing as before my illness.

In short, I was simply sluggish in body and mind.

It was recommended that I start a physical and wellbeing activity programme, but those that I researched seemed too regimented and excessive for my senior years.

However, in the first quarter of 2024, I commenced your exercise programme at Community Moves, Forestville.

Your programme, I thought, was better suited to the exercise routine I envisaged. That is, not to be too physically stressful. I didn't wish to become a bodybuilder!

Well, it quickly became very clear just how much my general condition had deteriorated.

So, I made the effort to attend your classes three times a week and found that the experience not only significantly improved my physical condition but also my mental wellbeing.

My weekly swimming capability came back to where it was before my illness, and, very importantly, I started enjoying life much more again.

I think the programme is great, as are the staff who guide you through the sessions.

The camaraderie with other attendees also contributes to a very enjoyable experience.

I am now continuing with the programme as part of my lifestyle, not just as a means of recovery, as in my case, but as a continuing activity to help keep me mobile and enjoying life.

SECTION 1: RESOURCES

1) PHYSICAL ACTIVITY AND LONGEVITY SELF-ASSESSMENT SURVEY

Take the **Physical Activity and Longevity Self-Assessment Survey** to assess your risk of all-cause mortality.

Instructions: Answer the following questions based on your typical weekly activities. Circle the option that best applies to you.

1. Aerobic Activity (Moderate-Intensity Exercise)

How many days per week do you engage in moderate-intensity activities (e.g., brisk walking, cycling, swimming) for at least 30 minutes?

(A) None
(B) 1–2 days
(C) 3–4 days
(D) 5 or more days

2. Aerobic Activity (Vigorous-Intensity Exercise)

How many days per week do you engage in vigorous activities (e.g., jogging, fast cycling, aerobics) for at least 20 minutes?

(A) None
(B) 1 day
(C) 2–3 days
(D) 4 or more days

3. Strength Training

How many days per week do you perform activities that strengthen muscles (e.g., lifting weights, yoga, resistance band exercises)?

(A) None
(B) 1 day
(C) 2 days
(D) 3 or more days

4. Sedentary Behaviour

How many hours per day do you spend sitting or lying down (excluding sleeping)?

(A) More than 9 hours
(B) 6–9 hours
(C) 3–5 hours
(D) Less than 3 hours

5. Flexibility and Balance Exercises

How often do you perform activities that improve flexibility or balance (e.g., stretching, Tai Chi)?

(A) Never
(B) Occasionally
(C) 1–2 days per week
(D) 3 or more days per week

Scoring Guide

For each question, assign points to your answers:

A = 0 points, B = 1 point, C = 2 points, D = 3 points

Add up your total score to evaluate your risk level:

Your Results

0–4 Points: High Risk
Your current physical activity levels may increase your risk of chronic disease and premature mortality. Consider incorporating more exercise into your routine to improve your health.

5–9 Points: Moderate Risk
You're doing some physical activity, but increasing your activity levels (especially strength and aerobic exercise) could significantly enhance your health and reduce your risk.

10–15 Points: Low Risk
Great job! Your physical activity levels align with recommended guidelines, contributing to better health and reduced risk of chronic diseases.

2) PHYSICAL ACTIVITY GUIDELINES PLANNING TOOL

For Universal Adult Populations (18–64 & 65+)

Purpose

This tool helps adults plan and implement weekly physical activity based on national and international guidelines. It translates broad recommendations into an actionable weekly plan that supports health, fitness, and long-term adherence.

Guideline Summary

Adults should aim for:

- **150–300 minutes of moderate-intensity activity per week**, OR
- **75–150 minutes of vigorous-intensity activity per week**, OR
- An *equivalent combination* of moderate and vigorous activity
- **Strength training at least 2 days per week**
- **Minimise sedentary time** and break up long periods of sitting
- Older adults (65+) should also include **balance and mobility** training several days per week

Weekly Planning Template

Use this template to build your personalised weekly plan:

Moderate Activity Goal: ______ minutes/week
Vigorous Activity Goal: ______ minutes/week
Strength Sessions: ______ per week
Balance/Flexibility Sessions: ______ per week
Sedentary Break Strategy: ________________________________

Daily Movement Targets:

- Steps/day goal: __________
- Incidental movement ideas: ____________________________

Example Weekly Plan (Universal Adult)

Monday: 30 min brisk walk (moderate)
Tuesday: Full-body strength training (45 min)
Wednesday: 20 min interval session (vigorous)
Thursday: Stretching/mobility + 30 min light walk
Friday: Full-body strength training (45 min)
Weekend: Optional active recreation (bike ride, swim, hike, gardening)

Behaviour Change Strategies

Use evidence-based behaviour strategies to improve adherence:

- **SMART goals** (Specific, Measurable, Achievable, Relevant, Time-bound)
- **Habit stacking** (attach exercise to existing routines)
- **Tracking progress** (steps, minutes, heart rate, sessions)
- **Social accountability** (classes, partners, challenges)
- **Reduce friction** (prepare clothes/equipment ahead of time)
- **Reward loops** (reinforce consistency and milestones)

Monitoring & Review

Review each week and record:

- Total minutes of moderate activity: ______
- Total minutes of vigorous activity: ______
- Strength sessions completed: ______

- Balance/mobility sessions completed: ______
- Longest sitting period: ______
- Sedentary breaks taken: ______
- Barriers encountered: ____________________________
- Wins & progress: _________________________________

Monthly Reflection

- What improved this month?
- What barriers still exist?
- What habits can be strengthened next month?
- What social/supportive systems can help you progress?

SECTION 2

PHYSICAL HEALTH

CHAPTER 5A

BREATHING

At this point, I also feel it's important to highlight the role of proper breathing mechanics and how these can affect our physical and psychological health. All the physical dimensions I discuss in this chapter are affected and influenced by breathing, as is the way we engage in all aspects of daily life. I've provided a simple overview of some of the science behind breathing mechanics, but if you would like to dive a lot deeper, there is a book called Breath, by James Nestor, that is unparalleled on this topic.

There have been many books that have impacted my behaviour, but I can't think of many that have had such long-lasting and notable impacts as James Nestor's book. One behaviour, in particular, has been life-changing, and that is taping my mouth closed when I sleep. I see your eyebrows raising, but bear with me. I've always had sinus issues. I had my tonsils out as a kid and was a snorer for most of my life. This meant that my default position to get the most oxygen in my system when sleeping was to open my mouth and breathe like a zombie all night, drooling over my pillow and waking anyone in earshot.

As I got more and more interested in anatomy and exercise physiology, and as the science around breathing mechanics started to permeate the fitness world, I did some upskilling on breathing training, and started taking more notice of my clients' breathing strategies, and also my own. At around the same time, I read Nestor's book.

Learning the differences between mouth breathing and nose breathing and the influence this has on a vast number of physical (and psychological) health measures was profound. One of these influences relates to the effect of breathing mechanics on our autonomic nervous system. Essentially, mouth breathing speeds our system up, nose breathing slows things down.

I'll leave the rest for you to read in his book, but for the last couple of years, I have been taping my mouth shut before I go to bed and breathing through my nose as I sleep. I wake up more refreshed, rested, and rejuvenated rather than feeling like I had a mini hangover every morning. I have now retrained my brain and don't really need the tape anymore.

I know the practice of taping my mouth closed when I sleep may not be recommended by Ear, Nose and Throat specialists, but it has been a revelation for me, especially in resetting my breathing strategy when I sleep. This may not be for you, and I suggest you consult your GP before trying it, but it was a worthy experiment for me.

Nasal breathing filters out particles, humidifies incoming air, and warms it to protect the lungs and improve respiratory efficiency. Additionally, research indicates that nasal breathing allows nitric oxide (NO) from the sinuses to enter the lungs and circulation which has established cardiovascular benefits [9].

There are three different dimensions of breathing. The biomechanical dimension, the biochemical dimension, and the psychosocial dimension.

The biomechanical dimension of breathing function refers to the neuromuscular respiratory pump. That is, how the nervous system and muscular system interact to influence and control our breathing. Good biomechanical breathing uses the diaphragm effectively and doesn't overly rely on the accessory muscles of the neck and upper thorax.

Primarily using the accessory muscles to breathe can cause a multitude of issues. Firstly, a weak and inactive diaphragm can result in poor postural and stabilisation strategies due to its connections to the spine and its important role in creating intra-abdominal pressure during activities that require spinal stability. This will be explained in more detail in the Stability and Balance section.

Additionally, say we take, on average, 25,000 breaths each day, and we are using the muscles of the upper back, neck, and chest to do so, rather than using the diaphragm. This is likely going to cause a lot of tension in that area. Headaches, jaw pain, and stiff necks are common in people who overuse their accessory muscles to breathe rather than the diaphragm.

The biochemical dimension of breathing refers to the effect breathing has on our blood chemistry. Usually, this is characterised by consistent hyperventilation, which means we breathe in excess of our metabolic requirements. The ratio of oxygen to carbon dioxide in our blood is then out of balance (hypercapnia), which can result in muscle tension, muscle fatigue, lowered energy-producing capabilities, and pain.

Unfortunately, hyperventilators often feel as though they are not getting enough oxygen, so they force themselves to increase their breathing rate, which simply compounds the problem.

The psychophysiological dimension refers to the relationship between breathing, brain function, the autonomic nervous system, and our mental/emotional state.

One of the most exciting advances in our understanding of breathing over the last decade or so has centred around our ability to use controlled breathing techniques to influence our autonomic nervous system. This is the involuntary nervous system that controls things like heart rate, blood pressure, and glucose metabolism, to mention a few.

The use of controlled breathing techniques has been shown to have positive outcomes on things like depression, anxiety, stress, cognitive decline and more. The yogis and Buddhists have been using these techniques for millennia; we are only just catching up.

CHAPTER 5B

STRENGTH & MUSCLE BUILDING

In recent decades, we've greatly increased our understanding of the role that skeletal muscle plays in maintaining health. Once thought of as simply a lump of tissue to move our bones around, it is now recognised as one of the most critical organs for healthy functioning. Note that I referred to our muscles as 'organs'.

Not only does the musculoskeletal system enable us to maintain our posture and physical function, and perform all our activities of daily living, but it also does so much more.

Muscle plays a large role in our metabolic health, storing blood glucose as muscle glycogen and aiding in the oxidisation of lipids (fats) and glycogen to produce energy [10]. The more active muscle tissue we have, the more efficiently we store and use nutrients.

Muscle works with other systems in the body, such as the nervous system and circulatory system, to help maintain optimal health. We'll look at balance in more detail a bit later, but our muscles' ability to interact with our nervous system is one of the key contributors to good balance.

Most notably, in my opinion, is its role as an endocrine organ, meaning it releases signals, called myokines, that communicate with other areas of the body to help maintain optimal function [11]. Only in the last ten years has this function of skeletal muscle become so widely recognised, and there is still so much more to learn, but it is actually incredible. For example, one of the signalling pathways from contracting muscle leads to an increase in Brain-Derived Neurotrophic Factor, which helps with neuroplasticity and neurogenesis [12]. These are good things for our brains. Very, very good things.

There are indeed hundreds, if not thousands, of myokines released by active muscle tissue, influencing processes like metabolism, inflammation, and cellular repair. This highlights why prolonged sitting is detrimental to health: no movement means reduced myokine release, which can impair these critical functions.

Why is it important for older adults?

If you've not yet heard of Sarcopenia, you should have, and if you have, you should be worried about it. Sarcopenia is the name given to the slow loss of muscle mass experienced as we age. Dynapenia is the loss of muscle strength, they are very closely related and equally important.

From the age of about 30, we begin to lose our muscle mass at a rate of about 5-10% per decade [13], depending on where you get your information. This loss of muscle mass accelerates rapidly beyond the age of 70 if left unchecked. Worryingly, the loss of strength occurs at an even faster rate.

For all the reasons I've detailed above, the loss of muscle mass and strength as we age is one of the biggest contributors to poor physical, mental, and social health for older adults.

Firstly, the loss of physical function reduces our ability to maintain activities of daily living, impacts our ability to engage in social activities, which then contributes to social isolation, and the spiral continues downward. Not to mention the increased risk of falls and injury associated with losing our physical capacities [14].

Poor muscle health leads to a reduced function of the other systems that are linked. Reduced nervous system function and blood flow, impaired tendon and ligament health, reduced bone mineral density and so on.

And as indicated previously, low muscle activity means low myokine activity. Essentially, we are taking our body from being a communication superhighway to delivering messages via a carrier pigeon. No offence to the pigeon, but this isn't great.

How can you improve it?

The good news is that you can improve your strength and musculoskeletal health at any age. The best, and most common, way to do this is through resistance/strength training.

Whether it be performing bodyweight resistance exercises at home or in the local park, going to the gym to use the machines and free weights, or joining a group class that focuses on strength development, resistance training needs to be a priority.

Activities like aqua-aerobics, yoga, Pilates, cycling and swimming are good, and provide a moderate resistance training effect, but the reality is that we need to be lifting heavy, pushing, pulling, and carrying heavy things a couple of times a week.

Variety is the spice of life. So, keep going to your yoga classes, and don't stop walking as much as possible, but also look for somewhere you can safely learn to load your tissues and provide the stimulus required to force adaptation.

Remember, no challenge, no change.

Now, before that little part of your brain starts telling you a story about why you can't do it — *my knees are no good, I've got too many health issues, my back hurts too much, gyms are for young people* — I'm here to tell you that's nonsense. No matter what you are dealing with, there is always an option out there for you and always a way to work around the majority of our common limitations.

You just need to commit to finding it.

The strength training guidelines for older adults are a minimum of two sessions per week. We like our members to come to a minimum of three, as that's where they tend to see the greatest benefit; any more than that and you're really cooking with gas. Just need to be mindful of pushing too hard, too soon, especially if you're starting from a low base.

You will be amazed at how just a little bit of strength training over a consistent period of time can change your life. Before joining Community Moves, Jennifer was scheduled to have foot surgery. The procedure was likely to reduce her pain but would also leave her with some serious mobility restrictions.

After just a few months of training with us, her pain had reduced so much that she cancelled the surgery and has never looked back. Just last week, we were talking about how she'd moved to a new home and managed to do most of the carrying of boxes and heavy lifting herself. She remarked that she'd never have been able to do that if she hadn't continued with her strength training.

You see, this is the thing. It's not just that she was physically capable of lifting the boxes and moving furniture around herself; it's the confidence that comes with regularly performing resistance training that convinces you that you are capable. "I can lift that, I've lifted heavier things in the gym…"

CHAPTER 5C

CARDIORESPIRATORY FITNESS

In 1953, Dr Jeremy Morris led an investigation into the relationship between physical activity and coronary heart disease (CHD) using London transit officers as his subjects [15]. The London Transit Officer Study was a seminal body of work that provided some of the earliest evidence linking regular physical activity to better cardiovascular health.

Morris compared the health markers of the largely sedentary bus drivers to those of more physically active bus conductors. He found that the drivers had nearly twice the risk of developing coronary heart disease and experienced more heart attacks than the conductors.

Since then, the links between cardiorespiratory fitness and health have been studied ad nauseam, with the same findings. Without fear of contradiction, we can say that if you have better cardiorespiratory fitness, you will be healthier and more likely to live disease-free, for longer.

Cardiorespiratory fitness (CRD) is a measure of the ability of the heart, lungs, and circulatory system to supply oxygen to the muscles during sustained physical activity and the muscles' efficiency in using that oxygen for energy production.

Why is it important for older adults?

Cardiorespiratory fitness is usually measured by testing someone's VO_2max, measured in ml/kg/min, which is the maximum amount of oxygen our body can utilise during maximal effort exercise.

Recording a VO_2max in the lowest range for your age is a more powerful predictor of all-cause mortality than other risk factors such as smoking, diabetes, and hypertension [16].

It is not so much about the number in and of itself but more about the work that needs to be done (or not done) to get to that number. For example, a 70-year-old man with a VO_2max in the high 20s or early 30s, putting him in the ‘very high fitness’ category, would have had to have undertaken regular activities and exercises that stressed his cardiorespiratory system over a long period of time.

It is the body’s reaction and adaptation to these individual and regular stressors that help improve its health and maintain a strong cellular and systemic environment.

During COVID-19, some of the worst outcomes occurred among people with the lowest levels of cardiorespiratory fitness. Studies consistently showed that poor fitness and low metabolic health were major predictors of severe disease, hospitalisation, and mortality—not just age alone. People with low fitness have a reduced ability to cope with physiological stress of any kind [17].

This same principle applies in other areas of life. Individuals with very low fitness often struggle to safely undergo surgeries requiring anaesthesia because their heart, lungs, and metabolic systems cannot tolerate the stress of the procedure or the recovery demands afterward. Low cardiorespiratory fitness is now recognised as a clinical risk factor in pre-operative assessment [18].

Even in everyday situations, the consequences are obvious. Travellers with limited fitness often find themselves unable to fully participate in tours that involve walking, stairs, mild hiking, or carrying luggage. Their bodies simply cannot meet the basic physical demands, meaning they miss out on experiences that should have been accessible and enjoyable.

Low cardiorespiratory fitness negatively impacts our health, our lifestyle, and our quality of life.

Whilst on the topic of cardiorespiratory fitness, I should also mention metabolic flexibility. Whilst VO_2max is a measure of the upper limits of CRF that primarily use muscle glycogen and blood glucose to fuel activity, there are also a lot of health benefits to being adept at performing for long durations at lower levels of intensity and utilising primarily our fat stores and blood lipids for energy. Being able to switch efficiently between fat oxidation and glucose oxidation, depending on the level of intensity of activity, is great for both metabolic and cellular health [19].

How can you improve it?

Before getting into the weeds a little on how you can improve your CRF, I'd like to tell you about a man by the name of Robert Marchand. In 2012, at the age of 100, Marchand set the 1-hour cycling record for his age category by covering 24.25km. He returned at age 105 in 2017 and set another record by cycling 22.547km in an hour.

During those years, between the ages of 101 and 103, it is reported that Marchand increased his VO_2max from 31ml/kg/min to 35ml/kg/min.

Robert Marchand died at the age of 109, and credited his longevity and vitality to regular physical activity, a healthy diet, and a positive mindset.

The body truly is an amazingly adaptive organism.

Improving your CRF is relatively simple in theory, but can be hard in practice. All you need to do is regularly get your heart rate up. The trouble is, it's uncomfortable. (Sensing a theme here?)

Luckily, you don't need to aim for an elite-level VO_2max like Marchand; in fact, some of the greatest improvements in health are seen when moving from the lowest levels of fitness to the next level up.

Walking is a great place to start if you don't do much of it. Then we look at activities like cycling, swimming, and jogging, where we can get a slow and steady increase in heart rate and maintain it for a period.

Finding activities that get you huffing and puffing and really stressing that system are the ones that drive your VO_2max up. These are best done by mixing intervals of hard work with intervals of rest, as trying to sustain high levels of effort can be very challenging and potentially counterproductive.

These can be difficult to perform if you're managing some musculoskeletal issues, but there are always options if you know how to work around your limitations or have someone who can help you do so.

It can be as simple as walking briskly up a steep hill and slowly making your way down several times, or as complex as performing sprints on a rowing machine. Different strokes for different folks. Excuse the pun.

CHAPTER 5D

STABILITY & BALANCE

'You can't shoot a cannon from a canoe' is a saying in the strength and conditioning world that illustrates the futility of having a lot of strength and power without having a strong and stable base to express it from. This concept rings true for anyone wanting to optimise their physical function and health.

When talking about stability, I am not only thinking of 'core' stability, which generally encompasses the area of the body between the ribcage and the pelvis, but am referring to stability throughout the whole body. Good stability requires our joints, muscles, nervous system, and brain to all work together to ensure we get the right balance between force creation, force transfer, and force absorption.

Speaking of balance, this particular aspect of physical functioning is of great interest to older adults and is a perfect example of how various systems work together to create stability. There are three main contributors that govern our ability to balance.

The visual system (our eyes) is the main player, as it helps us negotiate our immediate environment and provide instant feedback to the brain about where our body is in space and how we need to correct it if things go awry.

Then we have the vestibular system (our inner ears), which, simply put, helps to detect movements and the position of the head, and then provides feedback to the brain on our body position. This is why people suffering from disorders of the inner ear often experience vertigo.

Finally, we have the proprioceptive system (your nerves, muscles, and fascia) that relies on feedback from our neuromuscular system to tell our brain about where the body is in space. Try standing on one leg, barefoot, whilst closing your eyes. You'll likely feel all the muscles from your foot up through your lower leg start to fire up as they go into overdrive, working with your brain to keep your centre of mass in the best position to stay upright.

Balance is such a good predictor of longevity because it demands the seamless functioning of multiple systems — musculoskeletal strength, neuromuscular coordination, sensory input (vestibular/vision/proprioception), cardiovascular capacity and cognitive processing. If someone's balance is poor, it may signal early degradation in more than one of these interconnected systems.

In clinical cohorts, older adults with poor balance or slower gait speed faced a significantly higher risk of mortality over the following 8–10 years. Normative tests such as the single-leg stand (younger adults: ~40–60 s; older adults: markedly less) and the BESS show clear decline with age — making balance a practical early-warning indicator [20].

Why is it important for older adults?

The most obvious concern here is the link between balance and falls.

In 2019-20, the Australian Institute of Health and Welfare reported that approximately 133,000 older adults were hospitalised due to falls, with 50% of them fracturing one or more bones [21].

In 2021, the Australian Orthopedic Association National Joint Replacement Registry reported a total of 52,787 hip replacements,

68,466 knee replacements, and 8,733 shoulder replacements across all age groups in Australia [22]. Even if only half of these were performed on older adults, which is unlikely, it's a large number.

The scary part related to those figures is that many older adults can significantly lose their quality of life and increase their likelihood of early death after joint replacements [23].

These figures don't include the number of older adults who suffer from joint pain, injury, and falls but manage to stay out of the hospital. If they did, I'm sure we'd be looking at triple those numbers at least.

Without the ability to stabilise and control our body and balance both statically and dynamically, our risk of injury climbs. It is a classic case of use it or lose it. Just as I've talked about the body's ability to adapt positively to most stimuli provided, it will also cull any unused faculties that are taking up space and using energy.

So, if you've not been challenging your body to move in multiple directions, hop, skip, and jump, when you do accidentally clip the pavement and need a quick reaction from your feet to catch you before you end up flat on your face, the response from your body will be less than impressive.

Looking back at our evolutionary development, when we became bipedal and started walking everywhere, we had to develop a way of moving that enabled us to stay upright and balanced while using as little energy as possible. So, we stacked our head directly over our ribcage, which was stacked over our pelvis, with our weight falling directly below us, between our feet. As we moved, we kept our head upright and still, and learnt to rotate our arms and trunk in the opposite direction to our pelvis and legs. Walking and running are a beautiful combination of stability, movement, and balance that evolved over millions of years.

However, what happens when we fear falling? We drop our heads and start looking at the floor to ensure we don't get tripped up. This position of the head shifts our centre of mass and balance, pulling us forward, which actually takes us away from our most balanced position.

We also tend to start shuffling our feet, shortening our gait, and halting the swing of our arms. This moves us even further away from our most efficient, most balanced, and stable movement pattern.

We are no longer walking, we are essentially falling forward, each and every step.

How can you improve it?

There are a million ways to try and improve stability and balance. The best and most efficient way is to try and integrate more movement into your day, exposing your body to more situations that require a stability response. Simply standing more often than sitting is a good start.

When it comes to improving joint stability around specific areas of the body, a more targeted approach may need to be taken.

At Community Moves, we've always found that integrating specific stability exercises into our sessions, before moving into our primary strength-based movements, has been a great way to increase awareness, education, and joint function.

One of the first stops on the way to greater stability and balance is learning to create stability around our trunk without losing our breathing rhythm.

Have you ever seen footage of an Olympic Weightlifter fainting during one of their lifts?

It is not that the weight is too heavy or that they are not strong enough; it is due to a lack of oxygen to the brain. During maximal physical efforts, it can be very difficult to maintain normal breathing rhythm and, in fact, holding a breath and creating tension around the mid-section can help support our spine during a very heavy lift. In the case of the fainting athlete, the body is basically pulling rank and saying, "If you don't stop what you are doing and give me some oxygen, I will shut this party down and get it myself".

This is also the reason that people with hypertension, or those returning to exercise after undergoing some sort of cardiac incident, are advised not to perform exercises that require them to hold muscle contractions for extended periods, because we quite often hold our breath whilst holding a muscle contraction.

What we need to learn to do is breathe and create tension in the muscles around our abdomen and pelvis at the same time. This is what causes intra-abdominal pressure, which acts as a natural weight belt and stabilises our thoraco-pelvic canister (section of the torso from the ribs down to the pelvis).

This also ensures that we can perform activities that require a strong and stable base of support, whilst still supplying our working muscles and brain with the oxygen they need to function properly.

If you have good breathing mechanics and are able to use your diaphragm effectively, you'll notice that as you inhale, your abdomen will expand. This is not because you are taking oxygen into your belly but because, as your diaphragm pulls down to help the lungs fill with air, it pushes all the organs, blood, and soft tissues below it out of the way.

However, if you tighten up the muscles that support the abdomen, the lower back, and the pelvis (the 'core' muscles) whilst your diaphragm is pushing down, there is nowhere for all those internal organs to go, which creates intra-abdominal pressure.

Ideally, you should be able to continue to breathe using your diaphragm, supported by your accessory muscles when required, and maintain tension in your core muscles.

I often hear people talk about 'switching on' your core. I don't necessarily like this terminology as it implies that it is simply a case of being off or on. I prefer to think of the core muscles as a dimmer light. We can dial it up and create a lot of tension in anticipation of or reaction to a large force. Or we can dial it down and apply a smaller amount of stability to a less intense task.

Here's an exercise you can try to practice this co-activation concept:

Lie on your back with knees bent and feet flat on the floor.

Place one hand on your chest and one hand on your belly, then take some big, deep, diaphragmatic breaths, ensuring that it is the hand on your belly that rises and falls rather than the hand on your chest.

Once you have settled into your diaphragmatic breathing cycle, take the forefingers of both hands and walk them from the bony part of your pelvis, in towards your belly button, stopping about an inch away from the belly button on each side.

If you push your fingers from here in towards your spine, your lower abdomen should be soft and easily palpable.

Whilst pushing in towards your spine, perform a forced cough. The muscles you just felt push back against your fingers are your transverse abdominis (TrA) muscles, one of your deep-lying core stabilisers.

Now see if you can activate those muscles and push back against your fingers without coughing.

Here comes the challenging part.

Take a big, deep diaphragmatic breath, feeling that abdominal expansion, and hold the breath there.

Push your fingers back in towards your spine in the same spot as before and push back using your TrA muscles.

Now, exhale and try to maintain the same level of tension in your TrA as your diaphragm pushes up and reduces the amount of pressure in the abdominal cavity.

Continue for several full diaphragmatic breath cycles, trying to maintain the same TrA tension throughout.

If you managed to do this, you would feel the pressure build in your intra-abdominal cavity and would have successfully achieved co-activation of breathing and core stability.

If you lost TrA activation as you exhaled, keep practising this exercise until you can achieve at least three full breath cycles without losing control.

Once you have mastered this co-activation concept, you can apply it using the appropriate level of tension that any activity requires. As an example, carrying my 2-year-old daughter requires less co-activation than lifting either of my primary-aged sons. As I put one of them down and lift another, I dial up or down the amount of tension required.

In addition to the transverse abdominis and the diaphragm, the other main muscles of the trunk that support and create stable movement include the internal and external obliques, the rectus abdominus, the multifidus of the spine, and the pelvic floor. Think of the diaphragm and pelvic floor as the top and bottom of a can, and the obliques, TrA, rectus abdominus, and multifidus as the sides, front, and back.

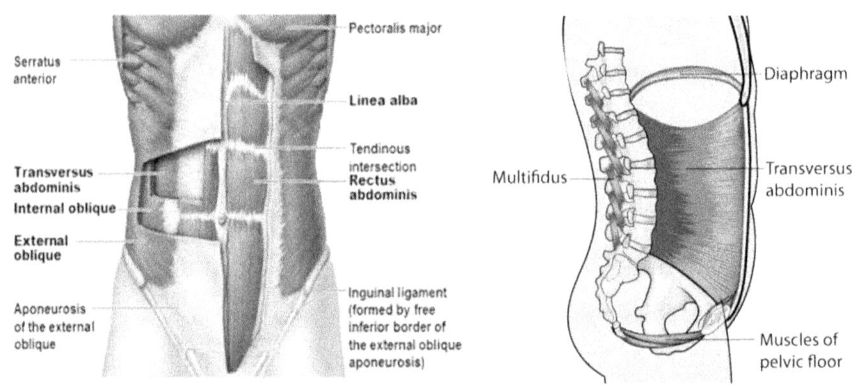

Frontal view of the muscles that make up our 'core'

Lateral view of the muscles that make up our 'core'

There are thousands of exercises and training techniques that target core strength. Pilates and Yoga are probably the best-known training methodologies that specifically address core stability, breathing, and postural control all in one. Each methodology has numerous training variations and formats.

In essence, any exercise that asks us to maintain 'core stability and breathing' whilst placing forces on the body that attempt to destabilise this area will force us to challenge those structures, and as a result, increase their strength, endurance, and capability.

For the relatively untrained or those returning to exercise after some time, walking straight into a Pilates or Yoga class may not be the best approach. Particularly if you are unable to get up and down from the floor easily, struggle to kneel for long periods, and haven't exercised in a while.

As good balance comes from multiple systems working together effectively and efficiently, it stands to reason that training balance needs to use a variety of techniques and modalities. Improved muscular fitness, improved core stability, improved coordination, improved neuromuscular communication, and more, will all help to improve our balance.

However, there are a couple of starting points and balance hacks that everyone can benefit from. Firstly, I would encourage everyone and anyone interested in not only improving their balance but improving their physical function overall to spend more time barefoot and engage in some specific foot strengthening and mobility exercises.

Our feet have a huge network of nerve receptors, similar to our hands, and are designed to provide a rich flow of feedback to our brains and body about where we are in space and how we need to react to the surfaces we walk on to maintain optimal alignment. Additionally, the fascia (essentially connective tissue) that runs under, around, and through the muscles and soft tissues of our feet actually connects up to our pelvic floor, diaphragm, and trunk musculature, helping to form a strong core and stable foundation for the whole body. This integrates with the breathing and core activation technique detailed above.

Before I outline some exercises that can help get the feet firing, I want to take things up to the eyes and something called the Reticular Activating System, or RAS for short. Once you understand how it works, you'll see how we can use simple eye exercises to switch it on — and how we can combine these exercises with our foot and core exercises for best outcomes.

Think of the RAS as your brain's filter and energy dial. It helps wake you up, keep you alert, and decide what information is important — kind of like a bouncer at the door of your awareness. It also plays a key role in controlling your muscle tone, which affects how stable, steady, and reactive your body is.

Why does this matter for balance? Because how tense or relaxed your muscles are — especially around your ankles, hips, core and spine — affects your ability to stay upright and adjust to movement. And the RAS helps manage that behind the scenes.

Here's the cool part: by doing targeted eye movement exercises like quick glances or smooth tracking, we can 'wake up' this system and send the brain the right kind of stimulation. This helps get your body into a more coordinated, responsive state — almost like turning on the engine before you drive [24].

It's a simple way to prime your brain and body to move better, and it only takes a few minutes. Check out the exercises in the resources section for details.

When it comes to stability and balance training, it is literally a case of learning to crawl and walk before you run.

As always, find someone or somewhere that can cater to your level of experience and makes you feel safe and well supported.

CHAPTER 5E

MOBILITY & FLEXIBILITY

I'll always remember the first time I went to China to meet my wife's parents for many reasons, most of which I won't bore you with now. However, one memory I'd like to share was witnessing my father-in-law preparing dinner. He grabbed a huge piece of beef and a large cleaver, took them out to the balcony, placed the beef on a chopping board, placed the chopping board on the floor, then squatted down into the deepest, most perfect squat I'd ever witnessed for someone his age, and proceeded to swing the heavy cleaver and dice the beef with surgical precision.

His expression of lower body mobility with upper body stability and coordination was striking, and not something that I was used to seeing with people his age, or in fact my age, in Australia.

I'm using the term mobility to describe the range of motion about a joint or multiple joints that we can control with stability, coordination, and strength. Flexibility refers to the range of motion that a joint or the tissues affecting a joint can be passively moved through, and it is one component of mobility.

One of the best comparisons we can make to illustrate what can happen to our mobility as we get older is to look at the movement of a toddler compared to a largely sedentary adult. Toddlers can sit down into a squat with their spine completely vertical and reach their arms directly overhead without so much as a wobble. Ask anyone over the age of 30 or 40 to do this, and you'll likely see some pretty interesting movement faults.

I can't remember where I read the following quote and have never been able to find the source (even google couldn't help!) but it's right on theme and too good not to share: "Of all the inventions which civilisation has invented for the torture of mankind... there are few which perform their work more pertinaciously, widely, or cruelly than the chair."

The body adapts to the positions that we expose it to the most. Muscles lengthen and shorten, some become tighter whilst others become slacker, tendons and ligaments stiffen or become more relaxed, and bones reform along new lines of force. Years of sitting in chairs, staring at screens, sinking into couches, and looking for comfort have stripped us of the requirement to regularly use our mobility capacity.

Our hips are tight, our upper backs are rounded, our shoulders are rotated inward, and our heads protrude forward. The scary thing is that I am seeing this posture more and more in teenagers and even younger children who spend too much time on handheld devices and too little time being physically active.

With the advent and advancement of running and fashion shoes came the loss of the mobility, strength, and function of our toes, feet and ankles. Arguably, feet are one of the most uniquely important areas of our body as a bipedal species. Loss of mobility and function at one joint simply means the forces it was designed to manage are passed up or down the chain. I believe a logical case could be made that holds the modern shoe, and a lack of focus on foot strength and function, to blame for many of the knee and hip issues we see in older adults today.

Thankfully, there are more and more companies now selling shoes that are actually good for our feet, and more health and exercise professionals are bringing attention to this key area of the body.

Good mobility starts from the ground up.

Why is it important for older adults?

Simply put, maintaining mobility helps ensure we can continue to access a wide variety of body positions, whilst performing activities of daily living, with a reduced risk of injury.

Let's use the rounded upper back position as an example. Say you've spent many years working at a desk, sitting in a slouched position with your shoulders internally rotated as you typed on your computer.

Over the years, the vertebrae in your spine have remodelled to adjust to this position, as have the soft tissue structures that help to hold everything in place. Your shoulders are now fixed in a forward rotated position, dropping down in front of a rounded upper back. To prevent you from looking at the ground and to ensure you get enough oxygen into your system, your head now sticks out in front of your body. The muscles behind your neck are significantly shorter and tighter than the ones in the front, as they work tirelessly to keep your head up.

Now, every time you reach up overhead to hang out the washing or take something from the top shelf of the pantry, you no longer have the shoulder and thoracic mobility to do so efficiently. As we have learnt, the body is pretty resilient and adaptive, so this lack of upper back and shoulder mobility doesn't stop you from performing the task. You just borrow mobility from somewhere else.

In this case, it's often the lower back that must hyper-extend to allow you to get those hands up overhead.

This may not be an issue right now, but as you get older and you perform these activities for the millionth time, with a body that's losing its strength, fitness, coordination, and mobility, you can be sure that a leak is going to spring somewhere.

We are all going to get injured or suffer from some joint or muscle pain at some stage. It's just part of the human condition. Regular exercise and physical activity aren't going to prevent all of these things from happening and may, in some instances, be the cause of the injury.

We'll never be able to quantify how many injuries or health issues we have prevented due to the benefits of regular exercise, but I'd much prefer to risk injury from moving a lot than almost guarantee it from moving too little.

How can you improve it?

One of the reasons resistance training is at the top of my list is that it is also great at stimulating and challenging many other components of physical fitness.

To perform many resistance exercises, you need to take your joints through the largest range of motion as you can manage with stability and control, whilst under load.

It is the regular movement of the joints through their available range that helps to improve their function. The cartilaginous structures surrounding our joints have a fairly limited blood supply and therefore require movement to flush nutrient-rich blood around the joint.

There is also a large neural component to our level of mobility, where the nervous system will essentially try to stop us from taking our joints through their full range because it doesn't trust that we have the stability or strength required to control that movement.

By frequently taking our joints through full range whilst under muscular tension and control, we are able to send messages from the tendons and muscles around the joint, back to the brain as a sort of 'situation report' from the field.

Static stretching is good if it makes you feel better. Combining load and mobility together is probably a bit better. Identifying your specific areas of most restriction and using soft tissue manipulation tools like foam rollers and massage guns to help release tension, and then trying to rebuild from there, is also a good start.

The reality is, though, spending ten to fifteen minutes a day on improving your mobility and then returning to the very same static positions that cause the issues for hours on end is akin to shuffling deckchairs on the Titanic.

Regular movement, including both structured exercise and incidental physical activity, is critical to maintain joint mobility and function. Understanding which activities and positions you regularly undertake that cause your major issues and finding strategies to address these can also be hugely valuable. Like using a standing desk rather than sitting all day, or spending more time barefoot rather than cramming your feet into sensory deprivation tanks (most common shoes).

Most of you will just shrug this idea off and call me sadistic, but for those who like a challenge, I want you to try and sit on the floor, for at least an hour, whilst watching TV at night for one week (not cold tiles or timber, I'm not insane). You will find that you have to constantly shift around to stay comfortable, which is good from a movement perspective, and you are challenging your joints, especially those of the lower body, to some ranges and angles that they haven't accessed for a while. Good for joint nourishment.

Additionally, you get to inadvertently practice getting up and down from the floor a couple of times a day.

After one week, do a bit of a self-assessment and see if any of it got easier. If it did, which I'd expect it would, you have changed something for the better. It doesn't matter what it was exactly or how it happened, but you shifted the needle. Try for a month now… and then two. Results come from consistency over time.

If you can't even get down to the floor, or have another barrier, obviously that's fine. Please don't do anything that is going to hurt you. The point is to try and change some of the habits that are feeding your lack of mobility and replace them with some that will improve it.

CHAPTER 6

JUDY

Judy is a remarkably strong woman. The reason I asked her to contribute to this book is that she is a great example of the power of a positive mindset and a never-say-die attitude. She has more excuses than most when it comes to exercise, but she doesn't let them get in her way. She attacks each day and each session with positivity, humour, and enthusiasm. This is Judy.

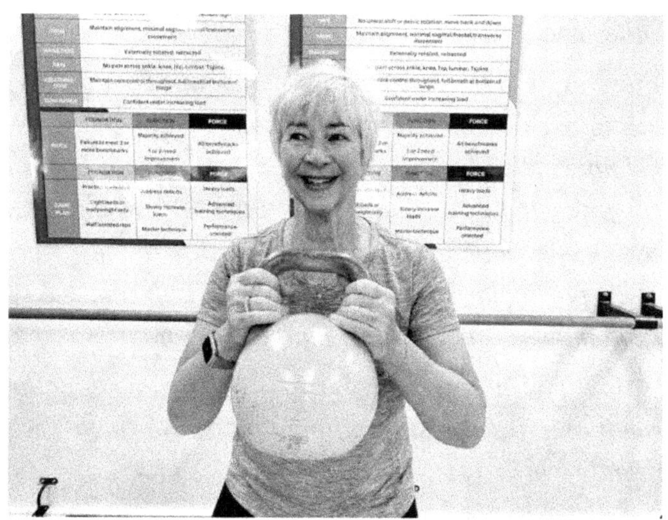

Judy working hard in the gym

I consider myself lucky, as I have always enjoyed exercising, and I raised my children to be the same. In my younger years, I regularly went to the gym and swam laps—about 1.5 km once or twice a week. I also rowed for around ten years in an eight and enjoyed this a couple of times a week.

My husband passed away 18 years ago at the young age of 59, and I was under considerable stress coping with this—managing businesses to carry on or wind up, and raising three daughters with their education needs. My doctors believed I internalised much of this stress, and in 2009, and again in 2012, I underwent knee replacements. My new knees have never really been "happy", but they have enabled me to walk. Sadly, they were done by different surgeons and are mismatched appliances, which has made my right side 11 mm taller than my left. I also battle with significant scar tissue around the knees.

After numerous ultrasounds, X-rays and MRIs, and experiencing complete instability when walking, I had my first of four spinal operations in 2014. I initially underwent a laminectomy, and during the surgery, a cyst was discovered in my spinal canal and removed. Exactly one year later, the pain returned, and I required a discectomy, during which another cyst was removed.

Why these cysts kept recurring was, and still is, a mystery. Due to the increasing scar tissue, surgeons could no longer perform these relatively simple procedures and decided that a spinal fusion would be required to prevent further cysts. This involved an eight-and-a-half-hour operation—a double spinal fusion with a bone graft and cyst removal. This particular cyst had integrated itself into the wall of the spinal canal and was especially difficult to operate on.

Four spinal operations later, I am left with radiculopathy, sensory changes such as paraesthesia and numbness, and motor weakness. I must constantly work to strengthen the muscles in my legs.

Prior to the spinal fusion, and because of my instability while walking (which I did a lot of), I had a serious fall in 2014. I shattered the ball joint in my left shoulder and broke my arm in four places, twisting my body in the fall to avoid landing on my knees. This required intricate surgery by a wonderful team, who inserted a rod with 17 screws into my shoulder and down my arm.

After that, there were no more operations for some time, but there was a great deal of pain. I was advised to explore all alternatives—physiotherapy, chiropractic care, pain clinics, dry needling, acupuncture and even marijuana oil. After several years of trying all of these, I was no better off and did not want to rely on medication.

Throughout this period, I continued working part-time, three days per week. Often, work helped take my mind off the pain. My employer invested in a Bambach saddle seat, which made prolonged sitting more comfortable. Standing was, and still is, more painful than sitting—movement is the best option.

I was searching for some form of physical exercise and a regular activity. I contacted several gyms and even joined one, but it didn't suit my needs. I also tried a Pilates studio, but after five private sessions, they advised that I shouldn't join a group class because I would "hold it up". In 2018, I came across an advertisement for Community Moves on my Facebook feed and immediately felt it was worth a try.

I retired in December 2019, and then COVID struck. No problem — I didn't miss an online class, with the help of a few simple purchases. I haven't looked back.

A structured class three times a week is perfect for me. Sometimes I can't do certain exercises, but the instructors are amazing, and I've learnt how to adapt movements to suit my needs. If something is painful, I don't do it — but I now find that I can do almost everything my gym buddies do, within reason.

There is a wonderful sense of camaraderie at Community Moves. You can be yourself and not worry if you need to adapt an exercise. Some people are incredibly fit with boundless energy; others are not. Everyone goes at their own pace and aims to do their best—or better than before. Many of us develop anxiety around certain movements as we move into our over-55 years, but this is something you overcome at Community Moves. The only person you really need to impress is yourself.

For a long time, I couldn't catch public transport on my own — buses, trains, ferries — it all became too overwhelming. I always kept a walking stick nearby. While I have always been a confident person, my mobility scared me. I couldn't even walk alone at Balmoral Beach, constantly worrying that I would trip. As I walked, the words "heel, toe, heel, toe" would repeat in my head. Now, I feel far more confident completing simple daily tasks.

Setting my alarm for 7 a.m. and bouncing out of bed to go to the gym three times a week is easy. Friendships have formed in class, and I've met many wonderful people to socialise with. There's always a chat after class, and often a coffee if time permits.

I describe the atmosphere at Community Moves as easy. The instructors are incredibly knowledgeable and generous with their time. The environment is ideal — there is space to move, adapt, and feel supported.

I prefer not to rely on medication for pain management. Sometimes it's necessary, but I've spent years on pills and worked hard to wean myself off them. With the right exercises, it is doable. When lifting weights, you are always given options. It's easy to manage injuries by adjusting the weight or equipment to suit your body. Over time, you improve and may lift heavier weights — but that choice is always yours.

In July 2025, feeling fit and well, I visited my GP for a routine annual check-up. Following the consultation, she advised me to see a cardiologist, as some of my results didn't "look good". I underwent the usual tests — a 24-hour heart rate monitor, a 24-hour blood pressure monitor and an angiogram. Within days, I found myself in hospital undergoing open-heart surgery — a triple bypass. One artery had a 95% blockage. There were no warning signs, no symptoms, no breathlessness — nothing.

Two weeks later, my cardiologist explained that I carry the Lipo(a) protein gene, which is completely hereditary. I am a non-smoker, drink minimal alcohol, am not overweight, and I walk regularly and train at Community Moves. It was a shock. However, the thoracic surgeon reassured me, saying, "You've been through so much already — you'll cope with this," which meant a great deal.

The first few days after surgery were difficult and frightening, particularly the breathing. Fortunately, Community Moves includes breathing exercises, which I immediately put into practice and felt they helped me cope. They say open-heart surgery is like a detailed engine overhaul for your body's most vital pump — getting you back on the road with a fresh start.

I began walking daily on flat, safe surfaces (quiet shopping centres are excellent for this). After four weeks, I attended cardiac rehabilitation, but only managed three sessions in the first week. I spoke with Van Marinos about returning to the gym earlier and completing my rehab there. I truly believe you must do what is right for you, and I felt comfortable working quietly in a corner of the gym, following the program with adjustments.

I am now five months post-triple bypass and feeling great. While I will need to take medication for peripheral artery disease, I feel like I am back — and thoroughly enjoying everything the gym has to offer.

My biggest obstacle remains getting down onto the floor and back up again. I've learnt how to do this (not always gracefully), but after years of being unable to, I am incredibly proud of that progress.

Kneeling exercises aren't possible for me, but alternatives — such as working on my back — are always available.

Lifestyle factors such as regular exercise, social engagement, mental stimulation and a healthy diet can positively influence cognitive function as we age. I couldn't imagine not exercising regularly. In retirement, many of us tick off bucket-list items — travel, caring for grandchildren, exploring local areas. A huge advantage of being at the gym is the stamina it provides to enjoy all these activities and keep up with everyone else.

I believe there are many men and women who need a little of this in their lives.

My neurosurgeon once warned me that I might not walk again. I persevered and achieved that milestone. He isn't worried about me anymore.

CHAPTER 7

STRENGTH & MUSCLE MASS FOR LONGEVITY

If you've made it this far, you should have a good understanding of why exercise and physical activity is so good for us. You'll also have figured that I, along with most other health and fitness professionals, place a huge amount of importance on maintaining strength and muscle function as we get older.

For the majority of older adults, starting a structured exercise program for the first time can be daunting, let alone going to a gym to start a strength program. Unfortunately, the health and fitness industry has traditionally not done a great job of catering to older adults. Older adults rarely see themselves represented in fitness advertising, and many mainstream gym environments can be intimidating and overwhelming.

If you're unsure of where to go and how to start, the best thing to do is to find a Personal Trainer, Exercise Scientist, or Exercise Physiologist who knows how to work with older bodies and people with a range of experiences and exercise backgrounds. They should know all of the stuff I'm about to outline and more, and will be able to take the thinking out of it for you.

Alternatively, you could try and find a gym like Community Moves. You'll get the added benefits of training with your peers and building social connections, whilst getting the technical coaching and support you need from an exercise point of view as well.

Either way, there are some concepts and aspects of strength and resistance training that are important to know which I've outlined below. After reading these, you might not be ready to start training like Mr. Olympia, but you should feel a little more informed and empowered when it comes to your own training.

Please note that any recommendations made here are general in nature and are extrapolated from the scientific literature. Additionally, this chapter is mainly focused on strength training. The other components of physical fitness should be included in your weekly exercise schedule and will have crossover benefits with one another.

The 'different strokes for different folks' adage always applies.

Terminology

Reps – The number of repetitions of a particular exercise performed consecutively.

Set/s – A group of consecutive repetitions (reps) of a specific exercise performed without resting. (e.g. performing 3 sets of 10 reps)

Tempo – The speed at which a single repetition is performed from start to finish.

The FITT Principle

Frequency (how often?) — 3x per week

The physical activity guidelines recommend older adults undertake two muscle strengthening activities each week. If you're starting from a very low base, this will be enough to start seeing some small changes.

If you really want to get some value out of it, I'd recommend undertaking some strength training at least 3 times per week.

Research has shown that performing around 10 sets per muscle group, per week, is the sweet spot for eliciting strength gains in older adults. If the goal is more about maintaining function as opposed to improving performance, you could get away with doing a bit less than that [25].

Intensity (how heavy?) — 6 to 20 repetitions, 3 to 4 sets, proximity to muscular failure

When it comes to increasing strength, heavier loads will generally produce the greatest results as there is a higher involvement from the neuromuscular system. These exercises can usually only be performed for 3 to 6 repetitions.

To increase muscle size, we generally try to choose a resistance that we can move for approximately 8 to 15 repetitions.

As with most things, there is a sliding scale, as muscle growth will also occur at lower rep ranges and muscle strength will also increase at higher rep ranges.

One of the more critical factors here revolves around a concept of 'failure'. This is when you can no longer perform another repetition due to muscular fatigue, or you need to stop due to technical failure, meaning you can no longer perform the exercise with the required technique.

For older adults, the goal should be to increase both muscle strength and size concurrently.

I would recommend using a resistance that you can do more than 6 repetitions, but no more than 20.

You should aim to perform a couple of sets of repetitions between 6 and 20, where you stop just a couple of reps shy of failure. Then, on the final set, perform a set to complete failure if you can.

Remember, the body responds to stress. Muscular failure is a great stressor and requires an adaptive response.

Type (what exercises?) — Key movement patterns, variety of exercises, speed training

Resistance training can take many forms and can be performed using many different pieces of equipment. Bodyweight training, resistance machines, free weights, kettlebells, sandbags, resistance cables, suspension cables, small children, large children; whatever it is, it doesn't really matter. As long as you are performing the exercises safely and there is enough resistance to stress the muscular system and drive an adaptive response, you're good to go.

What I would suggest is that you focus on key movement patterns and perform a variety of exercises, both single joint (like flexing/extending your elbow) and multi-joint (like flexing/extending your ankle, knee, and hip at the same time to squat), using different angles and body positions (standing, sitting).

These are the six key movement patterns I suggest you focus on: Squat, Hinge, Lunge, Push, Pull, and Carry. There could be an argument for Rotation to be included as well, but I would suggest that Rotation can and should be integrated with the other movements where appropriate.

You will also obtain a great benefit from including some impact exercises and speed training.

Without getting too nerdy, it is worth noting that one of the hallmarks of ageing from a muscle point of view is the loss of fast-twitch muscle fibres over slow-twitch muscle fibres. Our muscles have a mix of fast-twitch and slow-twitch muscle fibres that essentially govern whether that muscle is geared towards explosiveness or endurance [26].

As we age, and unless we do something about it, we will begin to lose the function of those fast-twitch muscle fibres long before we lose the function of the slow-twitch ones [27]. This is a problem because it's those fibres that are called into action when we need to move quickly to prevent a fall or react with speed to something. These fast-twitch muscle fibres are best trained and activated by either lifting heavy loads or performing our exercises with speed.

Extra caution should be taken when trying to add speed and resistance training together, as it requires a certain level of conditioning, coordination, and stability. If you haven't jumped or skipped since you were in school, then I wouldn't suggest you implement any jumping or explosive movements right away, as it will be too much for your tissues to handle.

Once you have been training for several months and have built up some capacity and confidence, you could start to slowly implement some of these more explosive movements. Things like jumps, hops, slam balls, and medicine ball throws are all good examples.

Make sure you are warmed up before you perform these kinds of exercises and that you are also not too fatigued to perform them correctly.

Time (how long?) — 45 mins to 1 hr

In order to address all of your movement patterns and get enough sets, reps, and rest in, I think you need at least 45 minutes to an hour for each session.

There are ways of shortening your sessions by combining exercises and working with less rest. This is called super-setting. We do this at Community Moves by having three exercises set up and having the group rotate around between each exercise with minimal rest. This helps produce a bit of a cardiorespiratory response as well as a strength response.

The scientific literature suggests that this method of training is less ideal for muscle growth and strength, as the shorter rest periods can detract from the energy and effort applied to each individual set [28].

However, our members tend to be less interested in squeezing the most out of each rep and more interested in maintaining their overall physical function and wellbeing. We implement elements of mobility, stability, strength, and cardio into most of our hour-long sessions, as for many of our members, the three sessions they complete with us may be the only bouts of exercise they do all week. It is our responsibility to try and improve as many aspects of their fitness as possible in as little time as possible.

For yourself, find what works for you and start there. For some people, simply performing a couple of sets of chair squats at home may be the best starting point, whereas others might enjoy getting to the gym every morning, six times a week, whilst also going hiking, cycling, and swimming at other times of the day.

Progressive overload

When beginning a resistance training program for the first time, changes in muscle strength and function can occur quite quickly. Most of these improvements can be attributed to an increase in the ability of the brain, nerves, and muscles (neuromuscular system) to work more efficiently together, rather than from an increase in muscle fibre size and power output [29].

The saying 'muscles that fire together, wire together', highlights the way that coordination of movement and muscle firing patterns can improve when regularly repeated.

Once the neuromuscular system has adapted and that initial change in coordination and strength has been attained, we need to ensure that we are constantly stressing and challenging our muscles. If we just stick to the same exercises, at the same level of resistance, working through the same range of motion, our bodies will adapt and then figure out a way to use less energy and resources to complete the task.

This is where the concept of progressive overload comes in. To match our bodies' increasing strength and muscle function, we need to continuously find ways to challenge them.

The easiest way to do this is to progressively add more resistance; however, you won't be able to keep doing this till you're eventually able to lift a car; it just doesn't work that way. We all have genetic ceilings, and only a rare few (think Olympians) have the capacity to exploit them.

So, if we can't keep adding weight infinitely, how do we progressively overload and challenge our systems? Well, here are a few ideas. You could increase the number of sets performed, reduce the amount of rest, increase the number of repetitions, increase the complexity of the exercise, increase the number of training sessions, perform two exercises for the same muscle group in a superset, and many more.

The main point is to ensure that you are always finding ways to keep challenging your muscular system. A good guide here is that if something feels easy, it probably is, and it may be time to find a way to increase the challenge.

You don't have to do this for every exercise in every session. Remember, this is a journey you should start but never finish, not a sprint. Pick one exercise each session that you want to focus on and find a way to increase the challenge on that one and that one only. Then, next session, choose another one.

Also, let's forget the old 'No pain, no gain' mantra — that's just stupid. If you are in pain, get help, and not every session needs to be bone-crushingly hard. There is still a lot of value in practising quality movement with synchronised breathing and stability. The goal should always be to keep improving and making small adjustments, but not at the expense of your overall health.

Perhaps we should say, "No challenge, no change" instead.

Managing limitations

I recently heard 'rehab' described as exercising in the presence of injury. I love this. Sure, there are some injuries and conditions that require a significant rest and recovery period, but, in my experience, the majority of injuries and issues people present with can be worked around. Exercise and recovery from injury do not have to be mutually exclusive. In fact, current pain management guidelines and injury management protocols encourage returning to some form of activity, however restricted, as soon as possible. Motion is lotion.

For a specific injury management program, find a good musculoskeletal clinician like a physio or sports chiro who is up to date with the research and adheres to a pragmatic return to exercise philosophy, and keep moving as much as you can.

I am a big fan of GPs and think they play a hugely important role in keeping us healthy, but many of them have not studied injury management or exercise science at the same level as other allied health clinicians. GPs studied medicine, and you should definitely see one when struggling with illness, but like all of us, they do not have all the answers to all the questions.

As an example, I recently had a member of my gym roll her ankle whilst walking her dog. She went to see her GP, who told her to stop walking and exercising for two weeks and to just rest as much as possible. This advice may have been the best available once upon a time, but nowadays it is totally out of step with rehab science.

Now, I'm not tarnishing all GPs with the same brush; I'm sure the majority would be more up to date with the science than this particular one and most would know to refer their patient on to a specialist in injury management. My point here is that injury doesn't need to equal inactivity, and there are plenty of professionals who can help you maintain your fitness goals whilst helping you return to optimal functioning.

When it comes to resistance training, we use the acrostic, GuideRAILS, to help manage any of our members' limitations. This can be applied in most settings and to most injuries.

R - Range of motion - Restricting or reducing the range of motion that we take a joint through can help avoid painful movements.

A - Alternate exercise - Select an alternate exercise that works the same muscle group or select a different muscle group altogether.

I - Isometrics - This is where you contract a muscle, but there is no movement at the joint and no lengthening or shortening of the muscle. This is a great strategy for rehab as it has also been shown to provide a pain-reduction effect.

L- Load reduction - Reducing the amount of load for a given exercise can help reduce the intensity of the exercise and assist with pain management.

S - Stability - Adding external stability by holding on to something stable or adding internal stability by activating stabilising muscles can help improve movement quality and reduce pain.

A 2008 study published in the Journals of Gerontology found that just ten days of bed rest resulted in a loss of nearly 1kg of lean tissue in the lower extremities and a 16% decline in muscle strength [30]. These findings have been replicated many times in different populations.

Protein

This is not a nutrition book. There is nothing quite like the world of nutrition, in which people are so wedded to one kind of diet or philosophy that they are willing to fight tooth and nail to protect and espouse its virtues, whilst simultaneously ignoring evidence to the contrary.

I think that some of the key problems surrounding the diet wars are that we are all different and absorb nutrients differently, we all have different food preferences and eating behaviours, nutrition research is expensive and hard to control over long periods of time, and much of the research is funded by big food companies that want to influence the results.

In saying that, luckily, there are a few things that have been studied ad nauseam and continue to provide consistent results (although I'm sure someone will still argue the fact). One of them, which is extremely important to strength and muscle mass, especially in older adults (hence my including it here), is protein.

Protein, or more specifically, the amino acids that make up protein, are essential for tissue growth and repair, hormone production, enzyme function, immune support, and overall metabolic processes.

When it comes to muscle strength, function, and maintenance, aside from resistance training, adequate protein intake is the biggest lever we can pull.

But many people are unaware of how much is needed and where to find it.

The Australian Dietary Guidelines recommend 0.6 to 0.8 grams of protein per kilo of bodyweight for older adults. This number was based on some pretty average studies that looked at nitrogen balance over the short term using only healthy young men. They were also testing for the minimum amount required to avoid deficiency, not what is needed to optimise function, maintain strength, and avoid frailty.

Considering that we become less efficient at absorbing and utilising protein as we get older — a process known as *anabolic resistance* — aiming for optimal rather than merely sufficient intake is crucial.

Leading researchers such as Stuart Phillips, Luc van Loon, and the international PROT-AGE Study Group [31] consistently recommend higher protein intakes for older adults, especially those who are active. Their research shows that consuming around 1.6 to 2.0 grams of protein per kilogram of bodyweight per day produces the best outcomes for maintaining muscle mass, strength, and metabolic health in ageing populations.

This recommendation is not arbitrary — it is grounded in multiple meta-analyses and expert consensus statements that highlight the increased protein needs of older adults.

I'm just standing on the shoulders of giants here.

So, a 75kg adult would need approximately 120-150 grams of protein per day. The best thing to do is spread it out over the day so that you are ingesting around 20-30g of protein per meal with some high protein snacks thrown in to top it up. This amount has been proven to initiate muscle protein synthesis, which is good, and slow muscle protein breakdown, which is bad.

I encourage you to do your own investigation and take a food audit to see how much you are getting; from what I've witnessed working with our members, most older adults aren't getting enough.

For example, I've had so many people tell me they eat an egg on toast in the morning to get their protein in. When I tell them that one egg contains only 6 – 7 grams of protein, I see the look of confidence on their face turn to shock and disappointment.

If you're not keen on eating 3 or 4 eggs for breakfast or changing your diet, which many find difficult to do, simply get a good quality protein supplement and fortify your existing diet with that.

The only real action here is to figure out how much protein you currently consume and then try to get that number as close to 1.6 – 2.0 grams per kilo of bodyweight as possible.

There are apps that can easily track this for you. I use MyFitnessPal, but there are many others out there.

The science of strength training and muscle building can be pretty overwhelming, as can the environments in which it often takes place. There are so many other bits and pieces we could go through here, but I don't want you to suffer paralysis by analysis.

Let's keep it simple. Find a good trainer or group exercise program, learn the technical basics and build a sufficient level of stability, coordination, and confidence. Then lift, pull, and carry heavy things, place your muscles and joints under stress, and move through different movement patterns consistently and over time. Don't stop for long periods, manage injuries as needed, get adequate rest and sleep, and consume the appropriate amount of protein.

I heard a great quote by Dr Stacy Sims that I'll end this chapter with: "Aim to be the oldest person in the gym, not the youngest person in the nursing home."

CHAPTER 8

RICHARD

Richard was referred to us in 2019 by a local chiropractor. He had a history of non-specific low back pain, had replaced a hip in his early fifties, and although he was quite active, he'd never really done much in the way of strength training. Richard is now the strongest guy in the gym. He pushes himself and trains with purpose every session. I owe him a lot, as he is the reason that the business evolved to include some more advanced sessions with heavier weights and higher intensities.

Richard has always been a great supporter of what we do, and I have always valued his input. He is kind, has a great sense of humour, and this is his story.

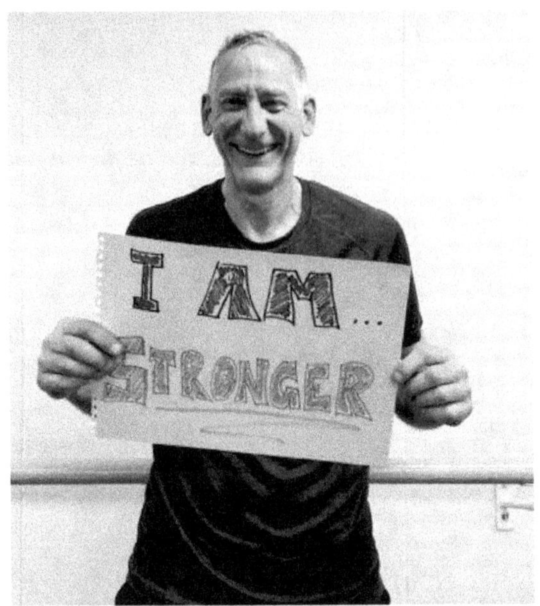

Richard happily engaging in one of our marketing campaigns

When I first walked into the gym six years ago, I was sceptical. Like many people, the idea of exercising in a gym wasn't particularly appealing — I've always preferred being active outdoors. However, joining Community Moves turned out to be one of the best decisions I've ever made for my health and overall wellbeing. Now in my early sixties, I'm stronger than I've ever been, free from acute pain, and generally healthier.

One of the biggest changes I've noticed is a significant increase in my strength. I've come to appreciate just how important weight training is for improving muscle tone, posture, bone density, injury prevention, and overall strength. Strength training is now a regular part of my routine — though it's worth saying that this didn't happen overnight.

Before joining the gym, I dealt with frequent bouts of acute pain, particularly in my lower back and joints. I was frustrated by the cycle of recurring physiotherapy visits, which ultimately led me to Community

Moves. Consistent, structured exercise has made a remarkable difference in managing and relieving those chronic pains.

Through a combination of stretching, mobility work, and progressive strength training, I've been able to reduce much of the discomfort I once lived with. Strengthening the muscles around my joints has given me better support and stability, reducing strain and helping prevent injury. Aches and pains that once felt inevitable are now largely a thing of the past.

Joining Community Moves has also helped me lose excess body fat accumulated over the years while building muscle. Regular training, combined with completing the Community Moves nutrition program, allowed me to rebalance my body composition and maintain weight loss. I'm far more mindful of what I eat and now focus on nutrient-dense foods — most of the time!

One of the unexpected benefits has been the social side. I joined primarily to improve my health, but I've formed genuine friendships that I wouldn't have made otherwise. It's a real community — coffees after class, daily messages, social events and clubs. And, as it turns out, peer pressure is a great motivator when you're heading to a 6 a.m. class in the middle of July.

The benefits didn't arrive instantly, and none of it was planned. When I first joined, the gym was smaller, classes were more limited, and the community was only just forming. I wasn't convinced of the value early on. But gradually, as I experienced the benefits of targeted exercise, I began joining the more challenging strength and cardio sessions as they were introduced.

To my own surprise, I now attend classes most days — and I can't see that changing anytime soon.

SECTION 2 - RESOURCES

SELF ASSESSMENTS

Breathing – The BOLT Score Test (Body Oxygen Level Test)

Purpose: Measures functional breathing efficiency and CO_2 tolerance.

How to perform:

1. Sit upright and breathe normally for a few minutes.
2. Take a normal (not deep) inhale through your nose, then exhale completely.
3. After exhaling, hold your breath and start a timer.
4. Hold until you feel the first natural urge to breathe (not until you're gasping).
5. Resume breathing through your nose and stop the timer.

Interpreting your results:

Less than 10 sec: Poor breathing efficiency (may indicate dysfunctional breathing or low CO_2 tolerance).
10 – 20 sec: Moderate function, but room for improvement.
20 – 40 sec: Good breathing function.
40+ sec: Excellent CO_2 tolerance and breathing efficiency.

Goal: Train to improve your BOLT score to at least 25 – 30 seconds, which is often associated with better endurance and reduced breathlessness.

Strength – 30 second Sit to Stand

Purpose: Assesses lower body strength, endurance, and functional fitness, especially in older adults.

How to perform:

1. Setup:
    - Use a sturdy, armless chair (seat height ~43 – 45 cm).
    - Place the chair against a wall for stability.
    - Sit with your back straight, feet flat on the floor, and arms crossed over your chest.
2. Execution:
    - Start a timer for 30 seconds.
    - Stand up fully and sit back down as many times as possible in 30 seconds.
    - Count each full stand (knees fully extended) as one rep.
    - If midway through a rep when time is up, do not count that rep.

Interpreting your results (average scores by age & gender):

Age (years)	**Men (avg. reps)**	**Women (avg. reps)**
60 – 64	14 – 19	12 – 17
65 – 69	12 – 18	11 – 16
70 – 74	12 – 17	10 – 15
75 – 79	11 – 17	10 – 15

Age (years)	Men (avg. reps)	Women (avg. reps)
80 – 84	10 – 15	9 – 14
85 – 89	8 – 14	7 – 12
90 – 94	4 – 11	4 – 10

Above average: Strong lower body function
Below average: Increased fall risk, reduced leg strength — would benefit from strength training

Cardio – 2 minute Step Test (2MST)

Purpose: Assesses aerobic endurance and functional fitness in older adults.

How to perform:

1. Setup:
   - Stand next to a wall or a sturdy chair for balance if needed.
   - Mark a spot on your thigh midway between your kneecap and hip bone — this is the height your knee must reach for each step.
   - Wear comfortable shoes and use a stopwatch or timer.
2. Execution:
   - Start the timer for 2 minutes.
   - March in place, lifting each knee to the marked height.
   - Use a steady pace, but you can rest if needed — just resume as soon as possible.
   - Count only the right knee lifts.

Interpreting your results (average scores by age & gender):

Age (years)	Men (avg. steps)	Women (avg. steps)
60 – 64	87 – 115	75 – 107
65 – 69	83 – 112	73 – 103
70 – 74	80 – 110	70 – 100
75 – 79	78 – 105	68 – 96
80 – 84	73 – 100	65 – 92
85 – 89	70 – 97	62 – 88
90 – 94	63 – 89	57 – 81

Above average: Good cardiovascular fitness
Below average: May indicate reduced endurance — would benefit from regular walking or aerobic exercise

Stability - Four Stage Balance Test

Purpose: Evaluates static balance and postural stability, assessing fall risk in older adults.

How to perform:

1. Setup:
    - Stand near a sturdy chair or wall for support if needed.
    - Wear comfortable shoes or go barefoot for better feedback.
    - Have a timer ready.

2. Execution:
   - Perform four progressively harder balance stances, holding each for 10 seconds:
     1. Feet together (side-by-side stance)
     2. Semi-tandem stance (one foot slightly in front, heel touching the other foot's big toe)
     3. Tandem stance (one foot directly in front of the other, heel to toe)
     4. One-leg stance (stand on one foot)
   - If unable to hold a stance for 10 seconds, stop the test.

Interpreting results:

Can hold all positions for 10 seconds → Good stability
Fails at one-leg stance → May indicate need for targeted balance training

Fails at tandem stance → Moderate balance impairment
Fails at semi-tandem stance or earlier → Increased fall risk

Mobility – Standing Toe Touch Assessment

Purpose: Assesses flexibility and mobility in the hamstrings, lower back, and calves, which are essential for functional movements like bending, lifting, and balance.

How to perform:

1. Setup:
   - Stand upright with feet hip-width apart and knees straight (but not locked).
   - Keep arms relaxed at your sides.

2. Execution:
   - Slowly bend forward from the hips, reaching down toward the toes.
   - Keep the back straight as long as possible before rounding slightly if needed.
   - Try to touch your toes (or beyond) without bending the knees.
   - Hold the furthest position for 2 – 3 seconds and then return to standing.
3. Measurement:
   - If fingertips go past the toes, mobility is excellent.
   - If fingertips touch the toes, mobility is adequate.
   - If fingertips do not reach the toes, measure the distance from the floor (in cm or inches).
   - Record the best of two attempts.

Interpreting your results:

Result	**Flexibility Level**
Palms flat on floor	Excellent
Fingertips touch toes	Good
5–10 cm from toes	Fair
More than 10 cm from toes	Poor

Notes:

If you experience pain or discomfort, stop the test.
Limited flexibility may indicate tight hamstrings, lower back stiffness, or mobility restrictions.
Stretching and mobility exercises can help improve results over time.

EYE EXERCISES FOR BALANCE AND COORDINATION

With core and foot integration

1. Saccades (Quick eye jumps)

Purpose: Improves rapid visual focus and engages attention and postural systems

How to perform:

- Stand tall or sit upright.
- Place two sticky dots (or thumbs) at eye level, shoulder-width apart.
- Keep your head still and flick your eyes back and forth between the two targets as quickly as possible for 10–15 seconds.

Progressions:

Level 1: Seated
Level 2: Standing in tandem stance (heel-to-toe)
Level 3: Standing on foam pad or balance disc
Level 4: Standing on one foot with **short foot activation** (foot tripod)
Level 5: Combine with **deep core engagement** (gentle brace and exhale during saccades)

2. Smooth Pursuits (Slow eye tracking)

Purpose: Enhances visual tracking and coordination between eyes, head, and balance systems

How to perform:

- Hold your thumb at arm's length.
- Slowly move it in an 'H' or 'O' shape.
- Follow the movement with only your eyes — keep your head still.

Progressions:

Add head turns in the opposite direction for challenge.
Perform while **balancing on one leg.**
Combine with **diaphragmatic breathing** (inhale during movement, exhale at completion).
Add **Toe Yoga** or **Short Foot Holds** during the drill.

3. Gaze Stabilisation (VOR Drill)

Purpose: Strengthens the vestibulo-ocular reflex (VOR) and supports postural reflexes

How to perform:

- Hold a letter or sticker at arm's length.
- While keeping your eyes fixed on the target, shake your head 'no' at a moderate pace.
- Perform for 10–20 seconds.

Progressions:

Use a metronome (goal: 120 bpm).
Stand on a foam pillow or an unstable surface.
Add marching steps in place or alternate hand touches to the opposite shoulder.

4. Near–Far Focus (Accommodation Drill)

Purpose: Enhances depth perception and visual control during movement

How to perform:

- Hold one thumb ~20cm from your face, and the other ~1 metre away.

- Shift your focus between the near and far thumb every 2 seconds.
- Perform for 30 – 60 seconds.

Progressions:

Perform in half-kneeling or single-leg stance.
Add ankle wobble cushion under foot.
Integrate with short foot exercise (*pushing big toe into the floor and lifting the arch of your foot*), core brace (*tightening your tummy muscles whilst maintaining breathing*), and nasal breathing (*breathing through the nose*).

ONLINE RESOURCES AND PROGRAMS

growstrongmethod.online

You can access a host of free and paid programs via the site above. However, if you're just starting out and want some simple exercise prescriptions, follow the programs below.

Home Strength Program

Here's a beginner-friendly workout plan designed for older adults, focusing on strength, balance, flexibility, and cardiovascular fitness. It's structured to be safe, effective, and adaptable to different fitness levels.

Frequency: 2 to 3 days per week
Duration: 30 to 45 minutes per session
Equipment needed: A sturdy chair, resistance bands (optional), light weights (optional). Can use household items as resistance – *such as water bottles, books, or a backpack with weighted objects in it.*

Warm-up (5 exercises, 30 seconds each, 2 rounds)

Warm-Up Video

Goal: Prepare the body, increase circulation, and reduce injury risk.

- March in place – 30 seconds
- Step & swing – 30 seconds
- Chest openers – 30 seconds
- Squats – 30 seconds
- Shuffle – 30 seconds

Strength training (2 to 3 days per week, 10 to 15 minutes)

Perform 1–2 sets of 10–15 repetitions for each exercise.

Lower body

- Chair Squats – Sit in a chair, stand up without using hands. Lower down slowly and repeat.
- Reverse Lunges – Hold on to the back of a chair, step back, and lower yourself down, keeping most of your weight on your front leg. Only move a small distance until you build your strength.
- Heel Raises – Rise onto toes, lower slowly. Can be done from the floor first, then progress to step if able.

Upper body

- Wall Push-Ups – Hands on wall, lower chest, push back. Lower slowly and repeat.
- Lateral Shoulder Raises – Lift light weights or water bottles up to shoulder height. Lower slowly and repeat.
- Bicep Curls – Lift weights toward shoulders, lower slowly.

Core & Stability (resistance band required)

- Anti-Rotation Hold – Stand side on to band attachment, hold handles out in front under tension. Engage core and breath at the same time. 3-5 breaths each side.
- Cable Front Hold & Slow March – Hold handle in front of face with tension on cable. Tighten core, breathe, and slowly shift weight from one foot to the other. 30 secs.
- Single-Leg Stance with Single-Arm Row – Stand on one leg or bias one leg with the other providing lighter support. Take the

cable or band in one hand and pull it in towards your ribcage using the arm opposite to the one providing balance. 10 each side.

Home Cardio Program

Cardiovascular exercise (3 to 5 days per week, 15 to 30 minutes)

Choose one:
Brisk walking – Indoors or outdoors, maintain steady pace.
Chair marching – Sit and march in place.
Water aerobics – Low impact, great for joints.
Cycling (stationary or outdoor) – Low resistance, steady pace.

Home Mobility Program

Flexibility & Mobility (daily, 5 to 10 minutes)

Controlled Articular Rotations & Neck Exercises

Neck, Shoulder, Hip, Ankle Joint Rotations – Focussed Neck Mobility & Strengthening

Cool Down & Breathing (5 minutes)

Deep Breathing – Inhale deeply, exhale slowly.

Progression Tips

Start slow and increase repetitions or duration gradually.
If balance is a concern, perform exercises near a chair or wall.
Listen to your body — stop if you feel pain or discomfort.
Stay hydrated and use active rest between workout days.

SECTION 3

SOCIAL AND EMOTIONAL HEALTH

CHAPTER 9

SOCIAL ISOLATION AND LONELINESS

For many older adults, not only does their physical health take a back seat for many years as they build a career and raise a family, but their social health can also suffer. Friendship networks grow smaller as people move away, lose touch, or no longer share the same interests. With retirement comes the loss of a whole network of professional and social contacts. Children grow up and have families of their own. Relationships end, and with them go shared friendships and acquaintances.

At the same time, the loss of physical function and confidence can often result in a slow withdrawal from social activities and outings, and thus, the proverbial snowball effect ensues.

From around the mid-20th century, there were a number of studies that looked at the impact of social isolation on rats and rhesus monkeys. The researchers consistently found that social isolation led to increases in stress hormones, increased anxiety response, reductions in neurogenesis and brain development, and more.

Decades later, research into the impact of social isolation on humans has unfortunately found much the same results. The evidence that social isolation and loneliness are significant contributors to depression, anxiety, and other mental disorders is irrefutable. If that doesn't scare you, then this should. In 2007, a group of psychology researchers from Chicago found that socially isolated older adults were twice as likely to suffer from dementia.

Demonstrating the link between mental health and physical health has not been as straightforward. However, a 2015 study published in the peer-reviewed journal, Perspectives on Psychology Science, by Julianne Holt-Lunstad and colleagues, did just that; they found that social isolation, loneliness, and living alone corresponded to an increase in all-cause mortality risk by 26-32%. This is comparable to smoking 15 cigarettes a day, with an increased risk of cardiovascular disease, stroke, and metabolic disorders [32].

In 2022 and 2023, I was fortunate enough to work with the ABC on a TV program called 'Old People's Home for Teenagers'. The basic premise was to see what would happen when a group of teenagers and a group of older adults spent time together, engaging in intergenerational activities and building friendships.

My role, as the 'Exercise Guy', was to help create and deliver some of the more physical activities and to assess the participants' physical fitness at the beginning and end of the series. Similarly, Dr Stephanie Ward assessed the older adults against a loneliness scale and other quality of life measures. For our older adults, both their physical fitness and mental health were quite poor.

My original exercise and physical activity plans had been quite extensive, as I really wanted to shine a light on the benefits of exercise (surprise, surprise). It wasn't to be, as one of the producers told me, "Watching exercise on TV is boring". So, in the end, we did a few activities that resembled exercise, but they were more tokenistic than functional.

At the end of both series, the older adults' loneliness scores and quality of life scores had improved drastically, as was hoped for, proving the mental health benefits of social interaction and connection.

And even though we hadn't done much in the way of structured exercise, there was an overall increase in the older adults' physical fitness scores as well. For five weeks, they had been getting in and out of buses, up and down from chairs, asked to walk from here to there, and had been provided a nutritious diet. Just living a more active, social, and balanced life, for a matter of weeks, had improved their health considerably.

Upon reflection, I realised that the social element of the experiment was the key ingredient. Because they were going somewhere, to do something, with somebody else, their whole outlook, sense of hope, and motivation to participate in life shifted.

It was a beautiful experience to be a part of and served as a great reminder to me personally about the importance of the social aspect at Community Moves.

Unfortunately, it was only an experiment that a handful of people were able to benefit from. The reality is that if it weren't for the show, the participants would have likely stayed in their rooms or homes, isolated, sedentary, and lonely.

There are varying statistics on the prevalence of social isolation and loneliness among older Australians, but it appears that somewhere in the region of 20% of them experience social isolation, with a slightly higher number experiencing loneliness, depending on where you get your information [33]. As much of the research in this area relies on qualitative data and self-reporting, it is hard to truly quantify the true prevalence of both. At the same time, we must also consider the variable nature of both experiences. Exactly how isolated and how lonely does one need to be before it starts to impact their health and wellbeing?

In researching some of the content for this book, I came across a story that resonated with this topic.

The Story of Anna and the Village That Forgot

In the early 20th century, in a small Italian village, there lived an elderly woman named Anna Maria. She had once been a central figure in the community, known for her cooking, storytelling, and wisdom. However, as time passed, younger generations left the village for the cities, seeking work and modern comforts. Many of Anna's friends passed away, and soon she was one of the last elderly residents remaining.

At first, villagers still visited her on occasion. But as their lives grew busier, the visits became less frequent. Eventually, people walked past her house without stopping, assuming she was fine or that someone else was looking after her.

Years went by, and one winter, a severe snowstorm hit the village. Roads were blocked, and people stayed indoors. No one noticed that Anna's house remained dark. When the storm finally passed, a young boy delivering bread knocked on her door. There was no answer.

When the villagers finally entered her home, they found Anna sitting in her chair, having passed away quietly, alone and forgotten. The fireplace was cold, her cupboards empty.

The entire village was devastated. They realised that, in their busy lives, they had neglected one of their own. The town's elders spoke of how Anna had once been a pillar of their community, and younger residents were filled with guilt for not checking on her.

In her memory, the village changed. They began a tradition where every family 'adopted' an elderly person, ensuring that no one was left alone again. This tradition continued for generations and became a model for nearby communities.

I have often had conversations with members of Community Moves about how they feel society has left them behind and how they, at times, feel invisible. Like Anna Maria, many have experienced the slow detachment from society as the next generation takes over. I'll always remember the sad visits to my grandmother when she was in aged care, walking past the TV room and looking in to see a row of bodies, almost lifeless, sunken into the chairs, not really watching the TV but rather watching time draw them closer to the end. Weak, frail, lonely and isolated.

I had never really thought much about the saying 'I'm dying of boredom' until then. Now it makes sense.

In the story above, the response of the town to 'adopt' an elder was a beautiful strategy to address the devastating experience of social isolation and loneliness. There are so many other strategies, formal or informal, established or unorthodox, that are rolled out every day to address these issues and many that address them as a byproduct. We'll talk about these and the power of social connection in the next couple of chapters.

CHAPTER 10

CYNTHIA

Cynthia was one of the first members to join Community Moves. During the early days, we would often have classes with just one or two people in them. You get to know people quite well when it's that intimate. Cynthia was, and is, always a joy to be around. Always supporting others, always checking in to see if you are ok, and always ready for a coffee and a chat if needed. She has expressed to me many times the joy and sense of belonging that she found with Community Moves and how she was becoming scarily withdrawn from society prior to joining. She has said that Community Moves saved her, but I think we ended up with the better end of the deal. This is her story.

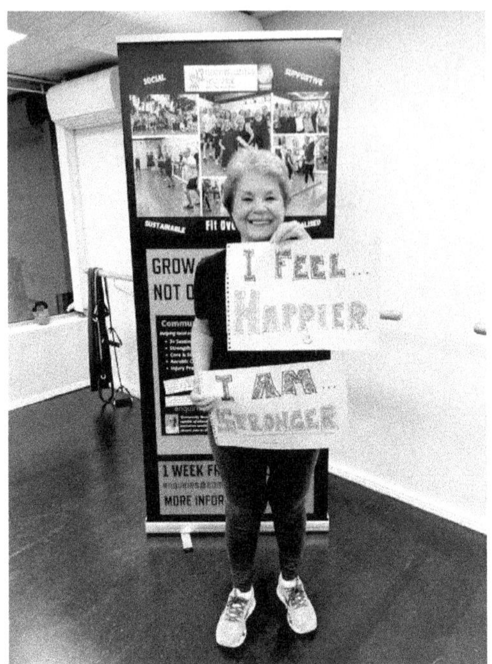

Cynthia joining in our 'I am..' campaign at CM Neutral Bay

My name is Cynthia, I am 73 years old and one of the original members of Community Moves Health & Fitness in Neutral Bay.

A bit of background about me. I am an only child, born in Australia, and raised on a Pacific Island in a loving family, although very protective, therefore sports activities were not on my curriculum. But who needed sports when you ran around all day with your cousins, and they were none the wiser what I got up to.

At 18, I came back to Sydney, which was a foreign country to me, i.e. language, way of life, but I quickly adapted.

I didn't start exercising until my late 60s after work, tried a few gyms but felt I didn't fit in (body, latest activewear, etc.), and you were shown the exercises once and no follow-up to see if you were using the equipment correctly. So, I gave up…

Then I was made redundant and started to worry about what's next, my work friends were still working, my married friends were busy with their grandchildren. I started to feel lonely, wondering what my future was going to be. I felt sorry for myself and became a couch potato for a while, then by chance, I came across an advert for Community Moves. I took a deep breath and decided to give exercise another go, and I haven't looked back

Van was very welcoming and explained what the gym was all about. I decided to give it a go, and I am still here.

Since being single, it has been the best decision I have made for a long time.

I made beautiful friends; we all go for coffees after class and socialise outside the gym, and we look after each other in times of need. I keep in touch with ex-gym members who have moved out of Sydney.

I attend classes 3 times a week, the variety of exercises has been good for my body, I am more flexible, I walk longer distances, my bone density is improving. And I have something to look forward to.

Community Moves has been a lifesaver for me; I'm so glad I saw that advert.

CHAPTER 11

POWER OF SOCIAL CONNECTION AND COMMUNITY

I never really understood the power of social connection and community until I started running Community Moves. To witness people's lives change in front of your eyes, as they go from experiencing relative social isolation to building a new network of friends and attending regular social gatherings, is an absolute privilege.

As a kid, I was pretty social. I never wanted to leave the party and always had a pretty good circle of friends around me. I am very close with my siblings and am lucky enough to have been able to share their circles of friends as well. Playing team sports was another opportunity to mix with people of similar age and interests.

It is only now, as a 42-year-old man with a family, that I have begun to experience feelings of social detachment. My friends are all at the same stage of life, focused on families, careers, and the daily grind. I have one or two close friends that I see semi-regularly, but am acutely aware of how quickly those relationships could suffer if we didn't actively work on them.

When I look at what is happening at Community Moves and what must be happening at any venue that delivers a shared activity to a specific group of people in a social environment, I understand why it is so powerful.

With regards to a group exercise program like ours, people initially attend because they are compelled to improve their physical health. They are then placed in a session with a group of people of similar age, from the local area, who share an aligned desire to improve their health. Just like the bad jokes we find in our Christmas Bonbons, people connect over the struggle of the exercises of the day, they share in the nostalgia of an old song, and find out more about all the things they have in common. This is before they go for a coffee.

Unlike me and my small friend networks, they don't really have to work too hard at it. They just need to turn up for their regular session, and the rest takes care of itself. The environment obviously needs to be accommodating, the formula can be relatively simple, and the positive outcomes to their mental health are almost immeasurable.

In John Arden's book, Rewire Your Brain, he details the positive effects of social interaction and how it affects your brain as well as many other areas of your body. The following list shows some of the many health-related benefits of 'social medicine':

- Decreased cardiovascular reactivity
- Decreased blood pressure
- Decreased cortisol levels
- Decreased serum cholesterol
- Increased immunity
- Decreased risk of depression
- Slowing down of cognitive decline
- Improvement in sleep.

I'm always interested in the root cause or evolutionary reason for human behaviours, biological processes, and physiological adaptations. My interest in our desire to be social and the manner in which this affects our brain and body is no different.

From an evolutionary perspective, I think it's fairly easy to understand. Our survival depended on us being able to work together to create shelter, find food, protect and raise our young, and pass on traditions and culture. In order for all of these things to have occurred effectively, we would have needed to build interpersonal relationships, show compassion and tolerance, build trust and loyalty, and experience the vast array of human emotions that come with collaborating with a group.

It makes sense that we're wired to seek the company of others. What I love is some of the neuroscience behind social connection and what is happening in the brain during group exercise. To highlight this, let's take a little peek into Anne's brain as she heads to her exercise session.

As Anne walks up to the gym and anticipates the positive social interactions she's likely to have, her brain starts to release dopamine, the brain's 'reward' neurotransmitter. This helps drive motivation and pleasure associated with socialising.

She enters the studio and is greeted by her fellow classmates as they wait for their session to begin. A mixture of men and women, ranging from mid-50s to mid-70s, on this occasion discussing the pros and cons of babysitting grandchildren.

This particular group have been attending this gym for 4 years and now form a close group of friends that have coffee together, go to the movies together, share photos on their WhatsApp group together, and support each other through all of their individual challenges.

Due to this social interaction and familiar connection, Anne's brain experiences a release of Oxytocin. Oxytocin, commonly known as the 'bonding hormone', helps to regulate our pro-social emotions, including trust, empathy, and more. Additionally, it has been linked to things like improved sleep and impulse control.

Once her class begins, Anne and her friends embark on a range of strength and stability exercises, contracting their muscles and moving their joints, sending blood flowing through their veins, and increasing their heart rate.

As Anne progresses through her exercise, the cells in her body start to activate some pretty amazing processes. During exercise, various genes related to cellular repair, metabolism, and energy production are upregulated, supporting overall health.

Through a series of cellular pathways that upregulate during exercise, Anne gets an increase in circulating Brain-Derived Neurotrophic Factor. BDNF plays a crucial role in supporting brain health by promoting the growth of new brain cells and strengthening neural connections, protecting against cognitive decline.

Additionally, whilst exercising, Anne's brain is increasing the production of neurotransmitters such as serotonin and norepinephrine. These hormones play a role in enhancing mood, cognitive function, motivation, and much more, even extending to other areas of the body.

At the end of the session, Anne and her classmates head for a coffee and a chat. Thereby reinforcing their connection, recovering from their workout, and letting all the body's internal processes work away to improve their physical and mental health.

Exercise-induced changes in your physical appearance, function, and capability may take some time. Changes in our internal biochemistry that improve our mood, cognitive function, and mental health happen immediately. When these events occur in our brain regularly, we put ourselves in the best position to live longer, healthier, and happier lives.

The internal biochemistry side of things is fascinating and extremely important to our overall health. However, there is more to it than that.

In 2008, a journalist by the name of Dan Buettner published a book called 'The Blue Zones'. Buettner identified the parts of the world that had the highest number of centenarians and then analysed their lifestyles, nutrition habits, and physical activity habits. He collated all of the data and found some commonalities between the groups that he attributed to their longevity. It's important to know that his findings were largely observational, which drew criticism from many on the research side of things, and he also went on to commercialise his work in many ways, which leads to a bit of bias towards his findings. His book was even turned into a Netflix series in 2023.

Putting all of that aside, there were some fascinating insights that are quite relevant to what we are covering in this book, especially in this chapter.

The more obvious contributors to longevity in these 'Blue Zones' were movement, good nutrition, stress management, and moderate alcohol consumption. I think most people would be able to look at those and go, yep, that's understandable.

The other few were not so clear initially, but once identified, they also make a whole lot of sense.

Having a sense of purpose, putting faith and family first, and having a strong social circle and sense of belonging were the remaining contributors to longevity, according to Buettner's Blue Zones.

We'll leave the sense of purpose and family first stuff for another time and focus on the theme of this chapter. What exactly is it about having a strong social circle and sense of belonging that helps us live longer? Once again, research comes to the fore to help identify some of the mechanisms by which regular social interaction and connection improve our health.

A 2010 study published in the PLOS Medicine Journal, by Julianne Holt-Lunstad and her team, analysed the results of 148 different studies, encompassing around 300,000 participants. An excerpt from the discussion links social relationships to a number of health-promoting factors [34].

> "*Social relationships are linked to better health practices and to psychological processes, such as stress and depression, that influence health outcomes in their own right; however, the influence of social relationships on health cannot be completely explained by these processes, as social relationships exert an independent effect. Reviews of such findings suggest that there are multiple biologic pathways involved (physiologic regulatory mechanisms, themselves intertwined) that in turn influence a number of disease endpoints. For instance, a number of studies indicate that social support is linked to better immune functioning and to immune-mediated inflammatory processes.*"

A study published in the Proceedings of the National Academy of Sciences of the United States of America (PNAS) in 2016, by Yang Claire Yang and associates from North Carolina, linked social integration to improved blood pressure [35].

Of particular interest, they noted that "*maintaining social connections in older adulthood plays a vital role in protecting health. Chronic conditions naturally increase during late adulthood as part of the ageing process. However, socially embedded older adults experience fewer disease risks, and our results from the NSHAP analyses suggest a causal role of social connections in reducing hypertension and obesity in old age. The deleterious effect of social isolation, in particular, was estimated to exceed that of diabetes, a well-known clinical risk factor for many chronic diseases including hypertension.*"

Ultimately, it appears that social connection and positive social relationships influence both our physiological and psychological/behavioural health in a positive manner. When we understand the role that isolation and loneliness play in upregulating our sympathetic nervous system and stress response, we can draw conclusions on how a reduction in this may improve our immune health, blood pressure, and other health-related biological processes.

With regards to its influence on our psychological/behavioural health, positive social relationships can influence our health behaviours by helping to promote healthy lifestyle choices. Community Moves is a prime example. It is the social side of things that fortifies people's adherence to the exercise. As many members have told us, they tried going to the gym alone or doing exercises at home, but it just isn't the same.

Additionally, positive social relationships can help to deter people from engaging in harmful lifestyle behaviours and provide support when 'falling off the wagon'.

Once again, this is not about promoting Community Moves but about sharing our experience and hoping to motivate people to find something similar that works for them. Not everyone is interested in finding new friends, building relationships, and increasing their networks, and that's perfectly fine. All we can do is present the evidence and provide anecdotes from our experience.

Our success lies in the combination of group exercise and social interaction, but there are many other iterations of the same theme. Below are a few examples of organisations that do the same thing. Although very different in our area of focus, the similarities lie in the purposeful and powerful combination of an activity with social interaction.

Men's Sheds

Started in Australia in the 1990s, the Men's Shed movement is now an international operation that seeks to support men's mental health, social connection, and wellbeing.

Book Clubs

There must be millions of book clubs around the world that bring people together regularly with a purpose and central focus. From what I hear about the book clubs that some of our CM members attend, there may be an even split between discussing a book and drinking wine. Excellent!

Sports Clubs

I still play football in a local over-35s competition. These days, it is just as much an exercise in mental and social health as it is about the actual game. There is something magical about team sports. Working with others to achieve a goal, understanding and accepting each others' strengths and weaknesses, and winning and losing together, all contribute to a sense of belonging and a social bond that is hard to replicate anywhere else.

Walking Groups

Similar to group exercise classes or the groups of MAMILs (middle-aged men in Lycra) cycling the streets every morning, walking groups are a great way to mix exercise with social interaction and connection. Walking offers a low barrier to entry to people who are just getting started on their physical activity journey and can be a great place to start building fitness and friendships.

CHAPTER 12

ANNIE

Annie is fun. An infectious smile and laugh, with kind eyes and big, fancy, blue-framed reading glasses. She is one of the organisers of our 'Foodies Group' and is what I imagine social connection would look like if it were a person. Everyone brings something different to a group dynamic, and all play their role, but you always need people like Annie, as they make the room brighter. This is Annie's story.

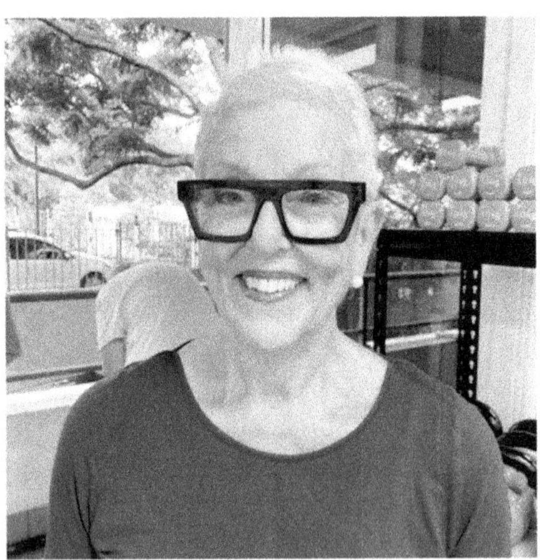

Annie always bringing life and laughter to our Community

I came to Community Moves nearly five years ago, just as I was turning 70. I had been divorced for many years and genuinely enjoy living alone. The divorce itself was difficult, and some family relationships were irreparably damaged, but I remain deeply grateful for those that endured.

I've always been fortunate to have a broad and varied network of friendships, along with many interests — reading, nature, snorkelling (I used to scuba dive), architecture and design, history, travel, philosophy, science, politics, food and entertaining. So when I made the plunge into Community Moves, I wasn't searching for social connection. I was simply looking for a supportive environment to achieve some health goals.

I had never joined a gym before. The pounding music, competitive preening and wall-to-wall mirrors held no appeal whatsoever. But the more I read, the clearer it became that to enjoy my later years, simply 'being active' and walking a lot was not enough. Retaining muscle mass, bone strength, flexibility and balance required a specialised area of expertise — one I would need to be taught and trained in.

I resigned myself to the idea of three one-hour sessions a week, assuming there would be a degree of boredom involved. What I didn't expect was that classes themselves would be the key. Exercising alongside others, being supported and supporting them in return, celebrating progress — both mine and theirs — turned out to be the magic ingredient.

The mood in the gym is consistently encouraging, supportive and unselfish. Meeting regularly, sharing the groans when we push ourselves, laughing together, and enjoying the very welcome coffees afterwards have created strong and lasting bonds. Friendship groups naturally formed, extending well beyond the gym — sometimes even travelling together.

With the introduction of social groups such as the Book Group, Movie Group and Foodie Group, that enrichment deepened even further. What began as a physical commitment evolved into something we genuinely looked forward to each week. The feeling of strength and physical capability in our bodies is amplified enormously by the delight of new friendships, shared experiences and a sense of belonging — an unexpected joy in later life.

Our later decades — our 60s, 70s and beyond — can be more complex than we ever imagined when viewed from the busy years of raising families, building careers, managing homes and running businesses. From a distance, retirement can look calm and leisurely. In reality, it often comes with unanticipated challenges.

Family dynamics shift, relationships fracture, careers end, children move away — sometimes overseas — and financial circumstances change. What can emerge, quite unexpectedly, are quieter, smaller lives, often accompanied by loss, disappointment or grief. Loneliness can creep in, and for many, it carries a sense of shame or personal failure that remains unspoken.

This is where a group-based activity like Community Moves becomes quietly transformative. The entry point is physical — many of us eventually realise that walking and golf alone are not enough for healthy ageing. Strong bones, muscle mass and balance require consistent, structured work. And that work needs to happen regularly, in supervised classes that prioritise safety and effectiveness.

Meeting three times a week becomes non-negotiable — and by definition, we are thrown together often. The environment is supportive, never competitive. Everyone understands that most of us carry injuries or limitations, and the encouragement of staff and peers permeates every session. We learn each other's challenges, celebrate progress, and naturally include one another — especially over coffee and conversation after class.

The social connections formed become an essential part of the week, though no one ever joins 'a club for the lonely'. Two years ago, this sense of connection expanded even further with the creation of member-run social clubs — Book Club, Movie Club, Walking Group and Foodie Group. These shared experiences, new outings and sense of belonging have enriched many lives in ways no one could have predicted.

Whether someone arrives with strong social networks already in place or not, the enrichment is felt by all. New members are warmly welcomed, effortlessly gathered up, and free to engage socially as much — or as little — as they choose.

Community Moves offers an evidence-based model that brings together all the elements we now know support healthy ageing. Its members are living proof that it works. Regardless of where you start, building a stronger body while feeling supported, understood and socially connected is a powerful enhancement of later life.

The phrase heard so often around Community Moves is, "Coming here has changed my life." Nothing could be truer. I only wish everyone had a Community Moves near them.

SECTION 3: RESOURCES

Check out the Loneliness Score, the Fear of Falling Scale, and the DASS-21 score below. These are good tools to use on yourself or give to a friend or family member to gauge where you are at and to see if you are at risk of becoming part of the 20%.

EIGHT-ITEM UCLA LONELINESS SCALE (ULS-8)

Instructions: Please indicate how often you feel the following statements are true for you.

Statement	**Never (1)**	**Rarely (2)**	**Sometimes (3)**	**Often (4)**
1. I feel in tune with the people around me. *(Reverse-scored)*	☐	☐	☐	☐
2. I lack companionship.	☐	☐	☐	☐
3. There is no one I can turn to.	☐	☐	☐	☐
4. I do not feel alone. *(Reverse-scored)*	☐	☐	☐	☐
5. I feel part of a group of friends. *(Reverse-scored)*	☐	☐	☐	☐
6. I feel left out.	☐	☐	☐	☐
7. I feel isolated from others.	☐	☐	☐	☐
8. I feel people are around me but not with me.	☐	☐	☐	☐

Scoring:

- **Reverse-score** items 1, 4, and 5 (i.e., 1 = 4, 2 = 3, 3 = 2, 4 = 1).
- Add up all responses (minimum score: **8**, maximum score: **32**).
- Higher scores indicate **greater feelings of loneliness**.

Interpretation & strategies:

Low loneliness (8 – 15): Maintain and strengthen connections

You have a strong social support network! Keep nurturing these relationships to maintain your wellbeing.

Strategies:

- Prioritise quality over quantity in your relationships.
- Engage in regular social activities that bring you joy (e.g. group exercise, book clubs, volunteering).
- Continue practicing gratitude and appreciation for the people in your life.

Moderate loneliness (16 – 23): Expand and deepen social connections

You may feel occasional loneliness or lack of deep connections. Strengthening existing relationships and making new ones can help. Strategies:

- Reach out to old friends or family members you've lost touch with.
- Join community-based groups (e.g. Men's Sheds, senior fitness classes, religious or cultural organisations).

- Schedule regular social activities (e.g. coffee meetups, group hobbies).
- Practice active listening to deepen connections and build stronger relationships.
- Use technology to stay in touch (e.g. video calls, social media, online forums).

High loneliness (24–32): Take action to reconnect

You may be experiencing significant social isolation. Prioritising social connection can greatly improve your mental and physical health. Strategies:

- Start small: Say hello to a neighbour or chat with a barista.
- Find structured social activities like a walking group, art class, or volunteering.
- Consider professional support — talk to a counsellor, therapist, or support group about feelings of isolation.
- If mobility is a barrier, explore phone or virtual connection programs (e.g. TeleFriend services, online community groups).
- Adopt a pet or get involved in an intergenerational program (e.g. mentoring younger people).

FEAR OF FALLING SELF-ASSESSMENT

Rate how worried you are about falling during the following activities:

Activity	Not worried (1)	Slightly worried (2)	Moderately worried (3)	Very worried (4)
Walking around the house	☐	☐	☐	☐
Walking outside on uneven ground	☐	☐	☐	☐
Using stairs (with or without handrails)	☐	☐	☐	☐
Standing on a chair to reach something	☐	☐	☐	☐
Walking in a crowded area (e.g. shopping centre)	☐	☐	☐	☐
Getting in/out of bed or a chair	☐	☐	☐	☐
Bathing or dressing	☐	☐	☐	☐
Carrying groceries or light objects while walking	☐	☐	☐	☐

Total score: Add up your scores (range: 8 – 32).

Low concern (8 – 12): Maintain strength & mobility

You have good confidence in your mobility! Continue to stay active and prevent falls.

What to do:

- Keep up with strength and balance exercises (e.g. Tai Chi, yoga, resistance training).
- Stay socially and physically engaged to maintain confidence.
- Ensure good lighting and clutter-free spaces at home.

Moderate concern (13 – 19): Build confidence & strength

You may hesitate with certain activities due to fall concerns. Improving balance and coordination can help.

What to do:

- Join fall prevention exercise programs like Otago or Stepping On.
- Practice balance exercises (e.g. standing on one leg, heel-to-toe walking).
- Use safe home modifications (e.g., grab bars, non-slip rugs).
- Walk with a friend or use walking aids if needed to improve confidence.

High concern (20–32): Reduce fear & regain independence

A strong fear of falling can lead to reduced activity, muscle loss, and greater fall risk. Taking steps to rebuild confidence is key.

What to do:

- Speak to a physiotherapist about a guided fall prevention program.

- Gradually increase activity with supervised movement (e.g., water-based therapy).
- Consider cognitive behavioural therapy (CBT) if fear is severely impacting daily life.
- Use assistive devices if needed — but focus on regaining strength and balance.
- Address environmental risks (e.g. install adequate lighting, remove trip hazards).

DASS-21 QUESTIONNAIRE

(Depression, Anxiety, Stress Scales)

Please read each statement and circle a number 0, 1, 2 or 3 which indicates how much the statement applied to you over the past week. There are no right or wrong answers. Do not spend too much time on any statement.

0 – Did not apply to me at all
1 – Applied to me to some degree, or some of the time
2 – Applied to me to a considerable degree, or a good part of time
3 – Applied to me very much or most of the time

1) I found it hard to wind down.
2) I was aware of dryness of my mouth.
3) I couldn't seem to experience any positive feeling at all.
4) I experienced breathing difficulty (e.g. excessively rapid breathing, breathlessness in the absence of physical exertion).
5) I found it difficult to work up the initiative to do things.
6) I tended to over-react to situations.
7) I experienced trembling (e.g. in the hands).
8) I felt that I was using a lot of nervous energy.
9) I was worried about situations in which I might panic and make a fool of myself.
10) I felt that I had nothing to look forward to.

11) I found myself getting agitated.

12) I found it difficult to relax.

13) I felt downhearted and blue.

14) I was intolerant of anything that kept me from getting on with what I was doing.

15) I felt I was close to panic.

16) I was unable to become enthusiastic about anything.

17) I felt I wasn't worth much as a person.

18) I felt that I was rather touchy.

19) I was aware of the action of my heart in the absence of physical exertion (e.g. sense of heart rate increase, heart missing a beat).

20) I felt scared without any good reason.

21) I felt that life was meaningless.

Scoring instructions

Each of the three DASS-21 scales contains 7 items, divided as follows:

Depression: Items 3, 5, 10, 13, 16, 17, 21
Anxiety: Items 2, 4, 7, 9, 15, 19, 20
Stress: Items 1, 6, 8, 11, 12, 14, 18

Add up the scores for the relevant items in each scale. Multiply the total by 2 to calculate the final score for comparison to DASS-42 norms.

Depression subscale		Anxiety subscale		Stress subscale	
Severity	**Score range**	**Severity**	**Score range**	**Severity**	**Score range**
Normal	0 – 9	Normal	0 – 7	Normal	0 – 14
Mild	10 – 13	Mild	8 – 9	Mild	15 – 18
Moderate	14 – 20	Moderate	10 – 14	Moderate	19 – 25
Severe	21 – 27	Severe	15 – 19	Severe	26 – 33
Extremely Severe	28+	Extremely Severe	20+	Extremely Severe	34+

This scale is intended for screening, **not diagnosis**. High scores may indicate need for further assessment by a qualified professional.

Seek and you shall find…

The last thing I want you to do here is research the various group activities and social clubs in your area. Check out the local library or council and see what they have on.

If you're on social media, look at some of the Facebook groups in your area and see if any interest you.

Go down to the local RSL or bowling club and check out the noticeboards.

If you don't ask, you don't know.

SECTION 4

IMPLEMENTATION

CHAPTER 13

THEORIES OF HEALTH BEHAVIOUR CHANGE

So, physical inactivity and social isolation are bad for our health, whilst regular exercise, particularly strength training, and positive social connections are good for our health. Seems straightforward, right? Wrong.

If everyone found it easy to exercise regularly, eat well, and maintain positive social relationships, we wouldn't need to spend anywhere near the billions and billions of dollars we do on healthcare. More importantly, individuals and families wouldn't have to suffer as much through their close ones' battles with illness and disease.

The reality is that health behaviour change is hard. There are so many factors that influence our lifestyle decisions, from those centred around our individual beliefs, the strength of our evolutionary biases, all the way through to the influence of government policy. Throw in the power and seemingly unlimited funds of industries like the pharmaceuticals and food manufacturing ones, and it's no wonder people find it so difficult to make healthy lifestyle changes.

This aspect of the human condition, our struggles with changing behaviour, have been studied at length. There are some useful theoretical models that can help us identify some of our individual and social habits, the impact of our local and global environments, and how all of these things integrate to influence our own behaviour. Plotting our journey against some of these theoretical models can serve as a good tool to help establish where we are in our own journey of health behaviour change and identify areas that we may need to manipulate to help tip the scales in our favour.

In this next section, I'll summarise a few of the models and provide an example for each of how I have seen these play out in real life with either Community Moves members, previous personal training clients, or family and friends. It's also worth noting that although we are looking at how these models influence the individual, they can also be applied at a whole organisation or community level.

The Trans-Theoretical Model (TTM), a.k.a. Stages of Change

The TTM or Stages of Change Model [36] asserts that in order for someone to change a behaviour, they must go through five different stages. Pre-contemplation, Contemplation, Preparation, Action, and Maintenance. In some versions, there is a sixth stage, which is Relapse, but as this can happen at any other stage so it is often left out.

Although a look at the model assumes there is a linear progression from one stage to another, it is quite often not the case. Some people will bounce between a couple of stages for a long time before moving to the next, and there is no guarantee that they will stay in any of the stages for any specific amount of time. Like human behaviour, the model accounts for fluctuations and fluidity.

Pre-contemplation is the point at which the individual hasn't even considered changing their behaviour. They may be unaware of the benefits associated with this new behaviour, be disinterested in changing their behaviour, or may simply be happy with the status quo.

Contemplation is when the individual starts to consider that a change in behaviour may be beneficial. Perhaps they've seen a change in their friends who have undertaken this new behaviour or have been advised by a health professional to consider making some changes. Whatever the instigator, they are now alert to the potential benefits of changing their behaviour.

Preparation is the stage where the individual begins to actively seek out information regarding the desired behaviour change and sets the wheels in motion to take that first step. They may be looking up different services and comparing different offerings to find something that meets their needs. They may be searching for articles and books on the topic to help them make a more informed decision.

Action. The individual has finally decided to act and has begun the new behaviour. They may have signed up for a new gym, started a new diet, quit smoking, begun a meditation practice… whatever! They have started, and they are filled with blind optimism, hope, and often more than a little trepidation.

Maintenance is the stage at which the individual has traversed the initial ups and downs of the new behaviour, and they've come out the other side. The new behaviour is now part of their identity and is hopefully there to stay.

Greg and the TTM

The first time I read about this theory, I immediately thought of one of my members at Community Moves, Greg.

When I opened my first studio, it was located on the ground floor of a small shopping arcade that had an escalator right in front of the studio entrance.

Greg used to take the escalators regularly, without even turning his head to see what was going on inside the gym. I'd then see him at the cafe around the corner, and we'd barely even share a glance. Greg was in the Pre-contemplation stage.

After some time, and as our membership started to build, Greg would traverse the escalator, but now with his eyes fixed on what was happening in the class. We gave each other a small head nod or a 'g'day' at the cafe. Greg was in the Contemplation stage.

Eventually, Greg came up to me whilst waiting for his coffee and asked about the service and what we do. He came and got a timetable from the studio, and we booked him in for a trial session. The Preparation stage was in full effect.

Greg attended his trial session and then signed up for a 12-month membership. He began attending Community Moves three times per week. Greg's strength, fitness, and coordination all improved as expected, but what was most pleasing and, I suspect, most important, was that he found a group of friends.

Greg has been attending Community Moves for almost five years now. He has had a few setbacks with injury and illness, as is par for the course with many older adults, and he's spent a bit of time away due to travel. The important thing is that Greg always comes back. He is in the Maintenance stage and continues to reap the social and physical benefits.

Health Beliefs Model

At a very basic level, the Health Beliefs Model [37] predicts that an individual's health behaviour will change if that individual believes they are at risk of harm, they can see the benefits to changing behaviour, and they have confidence in their ability to manage the behaviour.

The Health Belief Model emphasises how individual beliefs about health conditions shape health-related behaviours. It identifies several key factors influencing these behaviours, including **perceived susceptibility** (a person's sense of risk for illness or disease), **perceived severity** (belief in the seriousness of the condition and its consequences), **perceived benefits** (the advantages of taking preventive action), and **perceived barriers** (potential obstacles to action). Additionally, the model highlights the importance of **cues to action** (triggers that encourage behaviour change) and **self-efficacy** (confidence in one's ability to successfully take action).

Fay and The Health Beliefs Model

In the early days of Community Moves, I had a personal training client named Fay. She was an extraordinary woman. Intelligent, strong-minded, well-informed, well-travelled, funny, caring, and desperate to not let her 80-year-old body slow her down.

She had previously had a fall and knew that she was at risk of falling again (Perceived Susceptibility).

She was also aware that if she fell again, she might not be so lucky as to walk away with just a couple of bruises. The large majority of people her age who fall and break a hip never recover and are usually dead within five years (Perceived Severity).

Fay was very close to her family, especially her grandchildren, and wanted to maintain her independence and matriarchal status in her family. She knew that she needed to improve her strength and stability, and that a resistance training program was required (Perceived Benefits).

Fay had tried other gyms but came to Community Moves because we specifically catered to older adults and had created an environment that was welcoming, unintimidating, and supportive. We were relatively close by, and my availability suited her timetable (Perceived Barriers).

Before she signed up, she had seen some of our testimonials online and would often arrive for her session as one of our group classes was ending. She would witness the smiles on people's faces as they left and the positive impact we were having on these people's lives. This helped affirm her belief that she had found the right spot (Cues to Action).

Knowing Fay, I'm not sure there was ever a task that she felt she was unable to complete; she knew that she could improve her strength and refused to let her body influence her any other way (Self-Efficacy).

The Social Ecological Model

The last model we'll look at is the Social Ecological Model [38] of health behaviour change. This model posits that creating an environment conducive to change is vitally important in making healthy behaviours easier to adopt.

The model emphasises the multiple levels of influence, including individual factors, interpersonal factors, organisational factors, community factors, and public policy factors.

At the *individual* level, it is things like our values, beliefs, experiences, and personality that influence our behaviours. It is also our behaviours that can influence our beliefs.

At the *interpersonal* level, it assumes that we are influenced by, and have influence over, our social relationships, both good and bad, and that these relationships have a significant impact on our health behaviours.

Then we look at the *organisational* and institutional factors. What are the rules and regulations that influence behaviour? What is the culture like and the physical environment? How do individuals contribute to that?

At the *community* level, this model identifies the role that formal and informal social norms, local environments, and community engagement play in promoting or limiting healthy behaviours.

Finally, *public policy* also has a place at the table in this model as there is an undeniable influence that state and federal legislation can play in the management of health conditions and promotion of healthy behaviours.

Group Exercise and the Social Ecological Model

When someone joins a group exercise class, it's fair to assume that they inherently believe in the benefits of exercise. These beliefs are usually reinforced when they achieve certain milestones or overcome various challenges. Perhaps they have had a history of exercising and grew up with a family that enjoyed participating in sports and physical activity. Perhaps they have never exercised before but have come to realise that they need to do something to halt their current state of decline. *(Individual Factors)*

To state the bleeding obvious, people in group exercise classes are surrounded by other people who enjoy group exercise classes. They immediately have something in common and are engaging in a behaviour that promotes health. They are influenced by their classmates and vice versa. *(Interpersonal Factors)*

If the facility or gym they attend has a good program, an enjoyable atmosphere, a positive physical and social environment, and a wide range of times available to suit all lifestyles, then people are more likely to stick with it. *(Organisational Factors)*

If the group exercise class is designed to cater to specific populations or groups that share a number of characteristics (age, socioeconomic status, stage of life), then they are more likely to also build a cohesive community. Extending the connection of this community to the local area and engaging in activities that bring people together outside of the gym contribute to ongoing healthy behaviour. In this case, exercise. (*Community Factors*)

When it comes to the influence of public policy on an individual's decision to participate in a group exercise program, we may be a few steps removed. It's not as direct as something like the NSW Government's decision to mandate seatbelt wearing in the early seventies. Boom, instant health behaviour change. We are a little way from mandating exercise; however, things like government subsidies for individuals on Chronic Disease Management Plans to attend exercise sessions with Allied Health Professionals are a start. There are many examples of local, state, and federally funded programs that incentivise group exercise participation. This is where the influence of public policy lies in this model. *(Public Policy Factors)*

These models are just a few of many that can be used to help you learn about your own health behaviours and the many and myriad things that influence your lifestyle choices. Some of these may not be under your control; others may be. Either way, it's nice to know and kind of empowering… I hope.

I suspect I may have butchered some of these summaries, and there would be some academics in the area of health behaviour change that would have smoke coming out of their ears at the simplistic manner in which I've represented these models, but hey, I gave it a shot.

My biggest takeaway from researching and reading about these models is the important role that social connection and relationships play in influencing behaviour. I'm happy to be corrected here, but I don't think there is a single model that doesn't highlight its importance and influence.

CHAPTER 14

OK, I GET IT... HOW DO I GET STARTED?

Ha! I would actually be very surprised and extremely humbled to think that this book had such an influence that it was the catalyst for you to start a new exercise regime and find your social mojo. Truthfully, I don't expect that many will even read this outside of those who feel a sense of obligation, in case I ask them what they thought of it.

I'm fine with that. Being able to put my passion on a page and write about what I believe in is a reward in itself. And I'm proud of it.

If, by some miracle, you made it this far and this is the book you needed to read to serve as the springboard to better health and longevity, then read on.

I'm always wary of giving broad-brush advice when we are all so different, but I have been around the block enough times to feel confident that the advice below can be widely applied.

In terms of what your fitness regime should look like to support longevity, this will largely depend on your exercise history, available time, access to services, current physical condition, and a whole host of other influencing factors.

That said, here are 5 things you should consider when evaluating and planning your health and fitness regime to set you up for long-lasting success.

1) Is it enjoyable?

Simply put, we are a lot more likely to stick to something if we enjoy it. Some people bounce out of bed at the crack of dawn and head to a dark, sweaty room with pumping techno music for their morning spin cycle class. Others attend a quiet, peaceful Yoga session by the water.

To improve the likelihood that you will stick to your exercise routine for the long term, try to find exercise options that you enjoy and can see yourself committing to. Consistency is key.

2) Is it safe?

'If Youth Knew, If Age Could'. Freud pretty much hit the mark with this one. If we knew the toll that years of lack of exercise, poor form, and dysfunctional movement patterns would have caused our bodies as we age, we might have done things a little differently.

However, unless you were lucky enough to survive your adolescence and young adult years without causing any deterioration to the body, it's likely that you might be carrying a pre-existing injury or dealing with some form of chronic joint/muscle pain.

Regular exercise can help improve many of these issues and can greatly reduce the risk of further injuries occurring by helping to improve posture, balance, stability, strength, mobility, and so on.

To gain these benefits though, it must be SAFE. Australia's minimum standards to work as a trainer in the fitness industry are quite good, and there are plenty of ongoing professional development opportunities available. Unfortunately, this still doesn't mean every trainer is equipped with the skills and experience to deal with clients who have pre-existing musculoskeletal issues or are at risk of injury due to poor exercise history.

When selecting exercise options for longevity, ensure the staff are well trained and experienced working with older adults, look for classes or services that keep the number of participants fairly low to ensure you get the individual attention you need, and make sure to consult your doctor or allied health professional before beginning a new exercise regime.

3) Is it varied?

"I walk every day, so I don't need to do any of the aerobic sessions" is a comment I hear regularly when talking through our program at Community Moves. Now, don't get me wrong, walking is great. But it is just one form of exercise. It doesn't do much to improve your upper body strength and won't challenge the body through multiple planes of movement. How often, when walking, do you step sideways, backwards, cross your legs, jump, balance, turn, change pace and so on?

The human body is an extremely efficient and adaptive machine; if it isn't regularly challenged, it uses less and less energy and resources to perform the same task. It also has many systems that control movement and improve physical capacity. These all need to be exercised, or they will slowly deteriorate.

To keep us strong, mobile, fit, and healthy for the long haul, make sure your exercise program includes a range of aerobic, strength, and stability exercises for total conditioning. Things like balance, mobility, posture, breathing, and joint health should also be addressed to keep you learning and improving as you go.

4) Is it social?

We are social animals. Most of us enjoy things like team sports, spending time with friends and family, and sharing experiences with people of like mind. Maslow's Hierarchy of Needs lists our need for love and belonging right after our need for safety.

What I have learned from many of my clients is that their circle of friends and social network has slowly grown smaller over the years. Their children and grandchildren are off living their own lives, and for those in retirement, regular social connections can be very hard to maintain.

This is why our physical activity and fitness endeavours present a great opportunity to regularly connect with people over shared experience.

When planning your long-term fitness regime, try and find services that offer group classes, team activities, and actively promote a positive social culture.

5) Is it relevant?

The health and fitness priorities for many older adults are vastly different to those of younger populations. Athletic prowess, bulging biceps, and bikini bodies take a backseat to pain-free movement, injury prevention, and maintaining an active lifestyle.

Fitness activities that are going to improve your mobility so you can get up and down from the floor, increase your confidence to be able to chase your grandkids and pick them up safely, and enable you to lift your luggage up to an overhead locker without risking back and shoulder injuries are the type of programs you should look for.

'If you don't like something, change it. If you can't change it, change the way you think about it.'

If you haven't done much exercise in the past, start simple and work your way up. Seek the help of qualified and experienced personnel and engage in social exercise activities that improve your mental health as well as your physical health.

For those that already exercise regularly (well done!), check that your program has enough variety and flexibility to continually challenge you and promote improvements across all the body's movement systems.

It can be hard to start a new habit and to change a routine. The quote by Mary Englebreit above might help; it has often worked for me.

The Emotional Cycle of Change

Once you get started on your health and exercise journey, you will likely track along something known as the 'Emotional Cycle of Change' [39] (see figure).

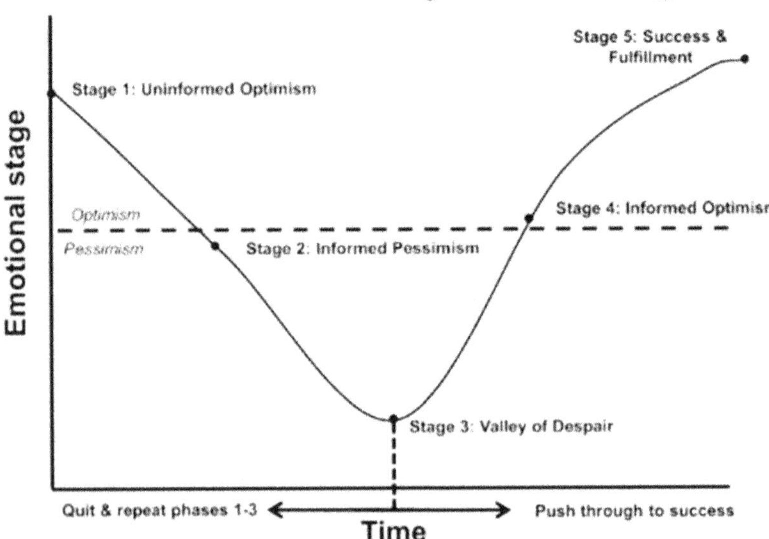

Visual graphic depicting the 'Emotional Cycle of Change'

In this model, after starting your new behaviour, you go from uninformed optimism to informed pessimism, to (my favourite) the valley of despair, to informed optimism, and finally to success and fulfilment. It is the 'valley of despair' that claims the most victims.

We see this in the fitness industry all the time. Someone starts a new program, and in the first few weeks, they are in the uninformed optimism stage. They are joyful, upbeat, confident, and filled with belief in their ability to stick to it this time. Then, after a month or so, they start to realise that consistency is hard, exercise can be hard, and the idea of doing it for a long time can be overwhelming. They have reached the informed pessimism stage. At this point, they may drop out, but most will persevere; however, they may have lost some of that initial 'joie de vivre' that they had a couple of months ago. They continue forcing themselves to attend, but their frequency, intensity of training, and commitment are wavering. They don't want to quit, but don't want to keep going. Welcome to the 'valley of despair'. This is where most people quit.

For those who continue and push forward, they are eventually rewarded with a new sense of optimism. Exercise has now become more of a habit rather than a chore, and the hard work is paying off. Beyond that, they are well and truly on the way to the success and maintenance stage, which is where the real magic happens.

At Community Moves, I can say without fear of contradiction that it is the social and community aspect that gets people through the valley of despair.

This is why it is so important that whatever you do, you do it with someone or in a group. You need to find other reasons to keep going when you're having that internal battle about calling it quits.

I was a volunteer Surf Lifesaver for a few years in my early thirties at North Bondi Surf Club and will never forget the group of old blokes that would meet at the clubhouse every morning at 6 am, trudge down the sand, no matter the weather, and swim across the bay. I'm sure there were mornings that they didn't want to get out of bed, but they didn't want to let their mates down and loved the coffee and banter afterwards.

Goal Setting

In Peter Attia's book, Outlive, he outlines this great concept of training for the Centenarian Decathlon. Boiled down, he identifies the things he'd still like to be able to do in his last decade of life, such as, get down on the floor to play with grandkids, carry heavy shopping bags up flights of stairs, pick a heavy object up off the floor, and so on, and then matches those activities with the physical capacities he requires now, in his fifties, to achieve them.

This is a great example of goal setting. His goals are relevant to him; they can be broken down into smaller, more specific goals, and they help provide motivation, both intrinsic (independence) and extrinsic (family).

Having a strong reason why you want to improve your health and maintain an active lifestyle is important. For many of our members, it is the desire to maintain their independence, to be able to take care of their grandchildren, to keep travelling the world, and to keep doing the things they love doing without their body letting them down.

Most of the goals our members tend to set are not performance goals, such as increasing the amount of weight they can deadlift or being able to perform 45 seconds of star jumps; their goals are generally related to the activities outside of the gym that are made easier by the work inside the gym.

This is where I advise you to start. Think of the things you would like to continue to do, or be able to do, for the next decade or more that require a healthy body, then look for an exercise program that will support that. As a general observation, most activities will require some combination of strength, cardiorespiratory fitness, mobility, and coordination.

If you are dipping your toes in the water for the first time, start small and go from there. When people begin their journey with us at Community Moves, we ask them to simply focus on getting here three times a week for the first month. They don't need to think of the three-month, six-month, or twelve-month plan, or what weights they are going to use and how our rehab and mobility programming syncs with our stability and strength components. None of that matters if they don't turn up.

Once you have begun something, anything, and have committed to it for a month, then you can start to think of the things that you would like to be able to achieve outside of the gym.

Is there a hill near your home that you haven't scaled for fear of physical incapability?

Do you take the lift instead of the stairs because you are worried about knee pain?

Is there a travel destination or tour you'd love to go on but don't have the physical confidence to take it on?

Do you get tired and frustrated with your lack of fitness when your grandchild wants to keep playing but you have to turn them down?

Find your why and let your exercise program support your goals.

The Power of Habit

Mahatma Gandhi once said, "Your actions become your habits. Your habits become your values. Your values become your destiny."

Performing an action for the first time requires planning and attention — from actions as simple as buying your morning coffee to complex actions such as reversing your car out of the driveway. As we repeat these behaviours over and over again, they require less and less conscious control and become almost automatic. They are now habits.

Charles Duhigg, author of 'The Power of Habit', writes about certain habits that have the power to influence the formation and strength of other habits; he calls these *'Keystone Habits'*. Duhigg uses many examples to highlight the power of these keystone habits, including that of Michael Phelps and his use of visualisation to influence his other gold-medal winning behaviours. From an early age, Phelps and his coach developed a mental showreel of the perfect race. He imagined the perfect start off the blocks, timing his final burst of speed with complete accuracy, and so on and so forth with detailed precision. From that point, prior to every race, Phelps closed his eyes and visualised that perfect race; this became a keystone habit. By doing this every race, it also ensured that his preparation became habituated, it ensured that his pre-race nutrition was timed perfectly and that his stretching routine became automated. Phelps had used a single habit to develop a whole range of habits that led to his incredible success.

Exercise acts in the same way as Phelps' visualisation habit. By turning up to the gym each day, or going for a run, or engaging in whatever exercise discipline works for you on a regular, consistent basis, exercise will become a habituated behaviour.

The question is, what other habits may be linked to regular exercise? This is quite subjective, but ask yourself this. Are you more or less likely to eat healthily after your exercise session? Are you more or less likely to feel good about yourself after exercising? If you are feeling good about yourself, are you more or less likely to engage in other healthy behaviours? This is the power of exercise as a keystone habit.

The difficult part is turning regular exercise into a habit. This is where we can enlist the help of another author, James Clear, who wrote the international bestseller, 'Atomic Habits', in 2018. James presents the 'four laws of behaviour change' as a framework for building new habits. The four laws include: Make it obvious, make it attractive, make it easy, make it satisfying.

I suggest reading his book as he provides some great detail on how to implement new behaviours or change existing ones. As a brief summary, using his framework to start your exercise behaviour might look something like this:

Make it **obvious** — *book your session the night before and put your workout gear on first thing when you wake up.*

Make it **attractive** — *Enlist the support of a friend and go together.*

Make it **easy** — *Find something close to your home to reduce the distance barrier.*

Make it **satisfying** — *Reward yourself with a coffee after class with friends.*

I think one of the best stories I ever read about using innovative ways to change habits came out of Sweden, where a train station installed piano keys as steps to encourage commuters to use the stairs rather than the escalators. It worked. They apparently recorded a 66% increase in stair use.

It's important to recognise that many of our habits have been entrenched for a long time, but it is possible to break them and create new ones. We just need to find the right inspiration.

CHAPTER 15

ANNE (MUM)

I started this book by writing about my father. It seems fitting that the final contribution was from my mother. She is an absolute force of nature. She religiously attends three or four gym sessions a week where she lifts heavy and moves gracefully, walks the dog two times a day, regularly takes care of her seven grandchildren (not all at once, but she could), teaches a singing group at the local community centre, has social lunches and drinks with friends, and is forever putting others before herself. Dad was my hero, but Mum is my guiding light.

She is an example of how to live well as we age.

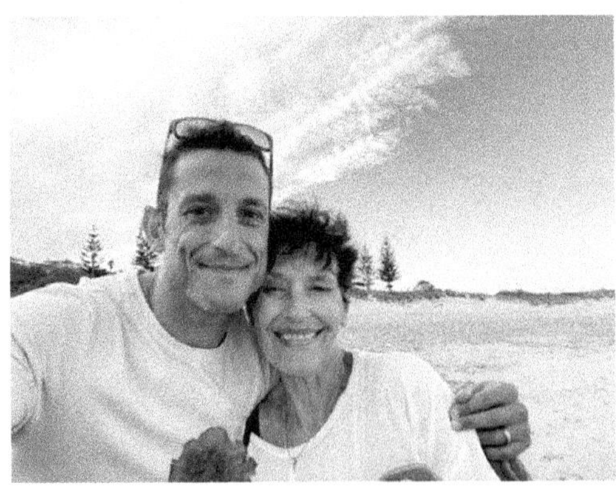

Mum and I having a selfie cuddle down at Curl Curl beach.

I grew up on the Northern Beaches in a very sports-oriented family. There was cricket, tennis, netball, football and swimming. My Dad played cricket and bowls and was an amateur boxer during the war. My Mum played tennis and in her later years, aqua aerobics, into her 90s. Her Dad, my grandfather, 'Dinny' Campbell, represented Australia in Rugby Union, defected to Rugby League and captained/coached Leeds in England for many years.

Living 5 minutes from Freshie beach, I swam. 5 am mornings lapping Harbord pool for the local swimming club, then came Synchronised Swimming; think a combination of Esther Williams and gymnastics. I loved it — I went on to become Australian champion when I was fourteen and remained so until retiring at 20, just prior to the sport being accepted into the Commonwealth Games. I was never a gym junkie, and in those days, exercise was always as a result of playing sport. Keeping fit and healthy was tantamount to achieving success in the sporting arena.

I went to NIDA to study Drama, where not only the skills of acting, voice and movement were taught but also the maintenance of a healthy lifestyle. Exercise and physical activity became part of my toolbox to ensure mental health, resilience, and stamina and the possibility of getting a job or not. Sadly, in the 70s, one's body shape could determine the outcome. I had been studying singing as a child and discovered a passion for Musical Theatre, one of the entertainment industry's most demanding disciplines. On tour for many weeks, dance and tap classes, yoga, and pilates were structured activities on offer for performers to maintain, hone or expand their skills. Throughout my 25 years in the industry and beyond I dipped into these activities, continuing jazz and tap classes with parents of my children's friends, coached my son's Soccer team and daughter's Netball team, intermittently attended Pilates classes at a local gym, played Netball until my ankles and knees screamed 'No More', and walked the dog/s.

Kids grew up, husband frantically busy, and I sought a new career in teaching students of Theatre and Screen Performance at Bankstown TAFE. Sitting in traffic for two hours per day, sitting on computers developing lesson plans, sitting at home marking students' work, studying, reading, keeping one step ahead of my classes, resulted in a sense of not being in touch with my body, exercise being sidelined, and my mental health rattled. I had been diagnosed with osteoporosis, and I needed to find a new purpose and a structured exercise regimen. Tried doing Yoga sessions online with Adrienne, but missed a class atmosphere, and I lacked the motivation to regularly commit to my lounge room floor. I went back to Pilates but needed more advice on technique, tried the machines, but again needed the motivation and moral support of fellow classmates. Meanwhile, grandchildren began arriving, and I wanted to be there. I wanted to run and play and dance and sing with them. Dropped work to 3 days per week and started to watch them grow and share the load with busy parents. Van was brewing a business idea, a realisation of his passion, an exercise program for over-fifties. He dangled that carrot before us.

We joined the Pilot program for 6 weeks at Norths Leagues Club, attended by a small group of interested over-fifties who were at similar stages of life and keen to live longer and be fitter. The three sessions per week seemed onerous, particularly for my husband, for whom regular exercise, bar walking the dog, was anathema. However, towards the end of the six weeks, our exercise sessions were becoming embedded into our lifestyle, and we were climbing those stairs more easily, our dog walks were less tedious, and our babysitting days were less exhausting! Friendships had blossomed with our fellow exercise mates, and the name 'Community Moves' was agreed upon. It was fun and we didn't want it to end.

In 2018 Community Moves opened at the Grove Arcade in Neutral Bay and my husband and I became committed, 3x per week, Community Moves junkies and our friendship network grew and grew. Our social calendar also grew. Health and nutrition workshops, rehab workshops, Barefoot Bowls, Trivia nights, Sips and Strokes, Xmas parties and then members bonding and connecting over coffee and dinners and outings and events. Covid threw us a curve ball and we despaired at a pending loss of muscle mass and forced isolation, but we were almost immediately participating in online Zoom classes, enabling exercise in our homes and the opportunity to chat to our friendship groups after our early morning sessions.

In 2022, despite the good news that my fitness levels, in combination with medication, had increased my bone density and decreased my risk levels for osteoporosis, I discovered that I was a candidate for a hip replacement due to osteoarthritis. I was at the peak of good health mentally and physically, so I continued my gym sessions, modifying exercises where there was pain and using the exercise bike to keep my hip busy. The op was a success, rehab was conducted at home and within four weeks, I was back at the gym, gradually rebuilding my mobility and balance and strength. Gym friends were so supportive and always there for me if I needed a walk or a chat or a coffee, or shopping done. Without my pre-existing exercise routine and fitness levels, and the supportive community around me, my outcomes would have been much worse.

In 2023, Lex and I climbed mountains and forded rivers in Scotland and Ireland, then returned home to his diagnosis of Stage 4 Lung Cancer. He believed that if he continued to exercise, he might extend the 6-month prognosis and even performed squats whilst the chemo infusion flooded his veins. He died on 13 September 2024, and our gym friends wrapped us in love and kindness and support.

My gym sessions keep me clear-headed, positive, strong, and connected. I am fit, strong, mobile, and healthy. I spend as much time as I can with my grandchildren and want to climb those mountains with them and be part of their future.

CHAPTER 16

WHAT ABOUT.....?

This chapter is a bit like the 'Frequently Asked Questions' section of an information leaflet. Over the years, there have been a number of questions and topics that have always bubbled to the surface, and below I have provided some short-ish answers to some of those common questions. I've probably had a million conversations with people about these topics, and my position has likely changed over the years as new and emerging research comes to the fore, but for now, this is where I stand.

Feel free to read the short answer only and skip the rest if you're looking for a concise response.

How much sleep do I need to get?
Short answer — Seven to nine hours.

There is a book by Neuroscientist Matthew Walker called 'Why We Sleep'. Read it. If you ever thought that six hours or less was ok or you were interested in the benefits of sleep and/or the risks associated with sleep deprivation, read it.

One of the things that Walker eloquently highlights is the fact that our requirement for sleep has been evolutionarily preserved. Meaning that, of all the changes that have occurred in our development over the whole period of evolution, our need for sleep has never been sacrificed.

There are so many deleterious physical outcomes that come from sleep deprivation, but the one that rightly scares so many people is the causal relationship between dementia and regularly getting less than six hours of sleep a night. Many people think they function well on six or less hours of sleep a night, and in many circles, it's even considered a badge of honour. Unfortunately, the more likely scenario is that they have simply convinced themselves that they function better on less sleep, whilst the chronic sleep deprivation is slowly causing a raft of physiological and psychological problems in the background.

If you do decide to read his book, beware, it may drive you to undertake some pretty radical changes in your sleep routine, so be prepared to be influenced.

There are a number of good sleep habit strategies out there. I like the '321' for its simplicity and ease of recall. I also try to give myself at least an eight-hour window for sleep each night. If I'm getting up at 5 am, I like to be in bed by 9 pm. I might read for half an hour before I nod off, but at least I know I'm in that seven-to-nine-hour window.

3 — Last big meal 3 hours before bed.

2 — Stop work 2 hours before bed.

1 — No screens 1 hour before bed.

What should I eat before and after I exercise?
Short answer — A nutritious, high-protein diet.

This is a question that I get often, and one that can have many different responses depending on the exercise you are doing and your personal preferences. For example, the nutritional demands of an endurance athlete are far different from those of a powerlifter.

When it comes to a general exercise program for average adults, not elite athletes, I think it is best to steer people to focus on getting a nutritious diet overall as opposed to targeting isolated meals and micronutrients. Our bodies have a large energy repository that, if well nourished, will have no trouble fuelling our workouts.

If we look at what's happening internally when we exercise, this can offer some additional insight into what may be required. When we are at rest, 20% of our blood flow goes to our working muscles, with the rest distributed in similar quantities to the brain, liver, gut, kidneys, skin and other regions. When we exercise, depending on the intensity, the working muscles require a significantly larger portion of the body's blood supply. During intense exercise, as much as 80 – 85% of cardiac output is redirected to the active muscles to meet their increased oxygen and nutrient demands. This redistribution occurs through vasodilation (widening of blood vessels) in the working muscles and vasoconstriction (narrowing of blood vessels) in less immediately essential organs like the digestive system and kidneys.

If you have a huge meal right before you perform intense exercise, the blood required to help digestion wouldn't be available, and that meal would sit in your belly, usually uncomfortably, until the exercise bout is finished. Even worse, your body may decide to get rid of it, and you may end up wearing the porcelain helmet.

If you don't eat enough or have enough energy stored in your muscles and liver, then you might find that you don't have enough in the tank to complete your exercise session with the intensity that you'd like. This can potentially lead to feelings of light-headedness and general fatigue.

My general advice is to stick to eating a nutritious, mostly wholefood, high-protein diet. Try not to eat a big meal right before you exercise; a simple carbohydrate snack like a banana or muesli bar might provide a little energy boost if needed. After you exercise, make sure your next meal contains a good source of carbohydrates to restore your glycogen stores and some protein to help cellular maintenance and structural repair. Oh… and don't forget to HYDRATE!

How come my balance hasn't returned yet?
Short answer — Because you don't train it enough.

This is one of those 'use it or lose it' situations. As we grow and develop from children to adults, we spend a lot of time running, jumping, climbing, riding bikes, playing sports and building our physical competencies. This is probably not reflective of childhood in 2025, but that's another topic altogether.

The point is that throughout these formative years, we are developing and enhancing the connection between our brain and bodies, with the ability to balance being one such example of this improved connection.

As we've established, the body will only maintain functions and structures that it needs and uses regularly. We get older, we play less, move less, and generally decondition. Balance suffers the same fate as many of our other physical abilities.

Performing three exercise sessions a week is good, more is better, but if those sessions only comprise a small amount of balance work, then the total time per week practising balance compared to the amount of time sitting down may not look so great.

The good news is, you don't have to stand on one leg all day — regular and consistent efforts to challenge your balance throughout the day will yield positive results. With the ability to balance being the result of a combination of multiple systems, it's best to challenge it in multiple ways.

Stand on one leg, stand in a tandem stance (heel/toe), and walk on a straight line. Add head turns and eye movements, close your eyes if you can, and even add other challenges like throwing and catching a ball.

One important point I regularly make is that although it may take some time to get your balance back, regular exercise will help reduce your risk of falling and will improve your ability to catch yourself or get up off the floor if you do.

Why is it harder to lose weight as I get older?
Short answer — Because you have less muscle mass.

Warning: This is a gross oversimplification of this topic and only delves slightly into the thermodynamics of energy balance and metabolism. Body composition is impacted by so many variables and is highly individualised. Seek the support of a dietitian or nutritionist before you embark on a weight loss strategy.

Muscle is a metabolically active tissue and therefore represents a significant contributor to our overall Total Daily Energy Expenditure. As we lose muscle mass, we see a drop in the amount of energy we expend.

If we maintain a similar diet in terms of energy input between the ages of 30 and 70, and we potentially lose 25% of our muscle mass, there is a slow and steady change in our body composition.

You may jump on the scale each day without the number changing, but internally you have slowly replaced lean tissue (muscle, connective tissue, bone, etc) with adipose tissue (fat). So, as you keep eating the same amount, your body is less able to utilise all those calories efficiently.

Quite often, people will then embark on severe dietary restriction and increase aerobic training in an effort to curtail their changing body composition. This can further compound the issue as they may lose weight on the scale, but this will also result in a further loss of muscle mass.

The key focus needs to be on increasing muscle mass rather than losing 'weight', and adding protein to the diet as well as fortifying it with nutritious, whole foods. For the body to lose fat, we need to be in a calorie deficit (less energy in than energy out) whilst working hard to maintain our muscle mass.

There are three main ways calorie/energy deficits are achieved. *Nutrient Restriction* is where you limit one kind of nutrient, such as 'Low Carb' or the 'Carnivore Diet'. By eliminating a whole category of food from your diet, you will generally fall into a calorie deficit. *Time Restriction* is where you manipulate the times at which you are allowed to feed. Michael Mosley popularised this with the '5:2 Diet'. There are other variations, such as the '16:8' or 'intermittent fasting'. All working on the basic premise that if we have less time to eat, we will eat less. Finally, you can implement some form of *Calorie Restriction.* Counting calories, mindful eating, flexible dieting, and portion control are all examples of how this can be done.

It is far better to be slightly overweight and strong, than weak and frail.

Does coffee dehydrate me?
Short answer — No.

I love coffee… in fact, I'm sceptical of people who don't. It's just so good on so many levels. I understand it's not for everyone, and that's fine, but I can't tell you the number of times I've heard someone say, "Don't drink coffee, you'll get dehydrated."

Caffeine is a diuretic, not a dehydrant. If you were walking through a desert, completely parched and on the brink of collapse, and the only thing you could drink was a coffee, you'd skull that thing like it was the elixir of life itself. The fluid content in that drink would be instantly absorbed by the body and cells to help return you to some level of homeostasis.

The small amount of caffeine in that drink will act as an antagonist to adenosine, which not only plays a role in sleep drive but also influences the kidneys to reduce urine output, amongst other things. Hence, influencing urine production.

If you maintain adequate hydration levels throughout the day, this will be insignificant in terms of the impact on your hydration status. Now, let's look at some of the known benefits of caffeine.

Caffeine intake has been proven to improve concentration and cognitive function, increase metabolism and fat oxidation, improve physical performance and enhance mood. It is not uncommon for athletes to use caffeine as a performance aid in many sports.

A single shot of coffee contains about 60mg of caffeine. General recommendations are that we consume no more than 400mg of caffeine per day, but this depends on the individual. Some are better at metabolising caffeine than others.

I routinely have a couple of double-shot lattes between waking up and midday. I try not to drink coffee too late, as it stays in the system for six or more hours and can impact sleep quality.

Moral of the story. Everything in moderation, and if you're dying of dehydration, drink the fluid that has a small amount of caffeine in it; you'll be fine.

Does alcohol make me fat?
Short answer — No.

Alcohol does not make you fat. I'm quite certain there are some skinny alcoholics out there. It does, however, contribute to your overall calorie intake, influences your nutritional behaviours, and messes with several systems that impact fat loss.

The next bit gets a bit technical, but stick with it, it's worth knowing.

Alcohol contains 7 calories (kcal) per gram. Just for reference, carbohydrates and proteins contain 4 calories per gram, and fat contains 9 calories per gram. One average glass of wine in Australia is 150 ml, and the alcohol content is around 13%. So 19.5 ml of that glass is alcohol. If 1 mg equals 7 kcal, then 19.5 ml equals 136.5 kcal per glass. The average bottle of wine therefore contains 682 kcal.

If I needed 2000 kcal per day to maintain my body composition, and on top of that, I drank a bottle of wine every evening, each year I'd be consuming an additional 249,000 kcal. In this case, I'd be very overweight and very ill.

Now, most of us (hopefully) don't drink that much, but when it comes to alcohol and body composition, its influence doesn't stop at the extra caloric intake.

Alcohol influences our food choices, restricts our body's ability to oxidise fat, impacts muscle protein synthesis, and reduces sleep quality, which creates a constant loop of hormone dysregulation, further affecting our body composition in a negative way. Not to mention the increased risk of things like Alcoholic Fatty Liver Disease and alcohol-associated injury or accident.

All that may sound scary, and it is, but keep in mind these deleterious effects come with a dose response. The heavier you drink, the more likely you are to experience the negative cascade of health issues. We must also consider the benefits associated with safe alcohol intake.

Every other Friday, I meet my best mate at a pub and have a couple of beers. We talk, joke, laugh, and feel happy and safe in each other's company. It's usually too late to get a coffee, and by the end of a busy week, beer makes a lot more sense. In this scenario, the benefits we gain are far greater than the negative effects of a small amount of alcohol.

There are many examples of situations where a glass of wine or a beer with friends and family might be just the thing you need to relax, reduce stress, and connect socially.

Like the saying goes, 'everything in moderation'.

Why do you make us do exercises with our toes and bare feet?
Short answer — Because they're critical to our overall function.

> *"The foot is the most complex piece of machinery ever designed."*
> *Leonardo da Vinci*

Think about this. We evolved over millions of years to be the only (full-time/obligate) bipedal mammal on the planet. We can walk/run huge distances, sprint short distances with explosive power, and hop, skip, and jump in every direction. Our feet evolved to enable us to do all of this and more.

There are 26 bones in each foot, meaning that 25% of the body's bones are housed below the knees. An extensive network of muscles and motor nerves is dedicated to your feet as well. One of our most important sensory input systems is the skin on the bottom of the foot. There are thousands of mechanoreceptors sensitive to light touch, texture, vibration, pressure, skin stretch and everything that's stimulated with every shift of the body and with every step we take.

As these different mechanoreceptors on the bottom of the foot are stimulated, specific muscle activation patterns are generated, which not only stabilise the foot and the ankle but also make their way up through the knee and hip, preparing the body to better absorb ground reaction forces for human locomotion. These ground reaction forces, and our ability to respond appropriately to them, are critical in endeavours of balance, strength, power, stability, posture, and alignment.

When we're in big, spongy shoes, unfortunately, a lot of these proprioceptors or mechanoreceptors are blocked or dampened. Shoes, and the lack of stimulation that results, can cocoon all of those bones and muscles and reduce sensory input. This limitation in foot muscle activity means limited circulation in the feet, circulation that is essential for the nerves, muscles, and skin of the feet and lower legs. Just think of what happens to a broken wrist when it has been in a cast for 6 weeks.

This is effectively what is happening when our feet are wrapped up in foam pillows day in, day out.

In addition to the lack of sensory and circulatory activity that occurs when shod, there is also the biomechanical and structural aspect to consider.

High heels, excessively cushioned trainers, and narrow-toed dress shoes can alter the structure of our feet and ankles, causing muscle imbalances, compensatory movement patterns, and malalignment.

I'm not suggesting that you throw out your shoes and turn into Fred Flintstone. Like any new concept or suggestion, it takes a while to get your head around. What I am suggesting is that you do a little of your own research, have a look at your shoes, have a look at your feet and ankles, and have a chat to your podiatrist if you have one (preferably one that also understands exercise science).

Try doing some of your physical activities barefoot. Buy a pair of minimalist shoes and swap them in every now and then. If you start to enjoy the feeling, you can try and slowly transition to them on a more regular basis. There will be an adjustment period. Your body will want to take the path of least resistance, so you will have to believe in the science and believe in your body's ability to adapt to new stimuli.

There are thousands of videos on the internet that detail exercises for improving the arches in the foot, the motor control of the toes, and the relationship between foot and ankle function and the rest of the body. Pick a few out, try them, and have some fun with them.

Why do we practice throwing and catching?
Short answer — It's great for the brain, and it's fun.

When was the last time you played throw and catch? Jumped rope? Climbed something? Kicked a ball? The majority of people will have to think back to their school PE lessons to answer this question.

All of these game-based activities that require coordination of the body and brain are brilliant for maintaining cognitive function and physical competency. The area of the brain that processes most of these functions is called the Cerebellum.

The Cerebellum contributes to a number of functions such as balance, spatial awareness, motor control and more. When we consider the role that all of these play in falls prevention and postural control, practising things that challenge and train our Cerebellum makes sense.

Additionally, when you get a group of people together that haven't done something like this for a long while, aside from the initial feelings of trepidation and confusion, by the end of the exercise, the overwhelming mood is one of fun and laughter.

For some people, this may also be the only time of day when they get a chance to smile and connect with someone.

If you don't have anyone to play with, you can still get the coordination benefits by standing a metre away from a wall and playing throw and catch with yourself. Try throwing with your right and catching with your left. Challenge yourself by seeing how many times you catch the ball in a minute or stand on one leg, and combine balance training as well.

Never stop playing. Good for the body, and good for the soul.

Why do we finish each session with a couple of minutes of quiet breathing? Short answer — Stress reduction and systemic recovery.

As I touched on earlier in the book, slow, controlled breathing was once considered a practice limited to Buddhist Monks, Yogis, and hippies. Over the last couple of decades, this has changed drastically with breathing exercises prescribed to everyone from high-flying executives and elite athletes to the average Joe Blow who's looking to control his anxiety.

This seismic shift in popularity has been led by science, anchored by the discovery of our ability to influence our autonomic nervous system (ANS). The ANS is responsible for slowing our internal processes down and speeding them up when required, all the while acting without conscious control.

For example, when we exercise, our sympathetic nervous system responds to this stressor by increasing heart rate, increasing blood pressure, shunting blood to working muscles and away from other organs, and releasing a number of inflammatory cytokines. When we go to sleep, our parasympathetic nervous system slows everything down. Our heart rate slows, our body temperature cools, and the many processes of cellular building and recovery take place.

When our sympathetic nervous system is placed in overdrive due to the millions of other stressors we encounter, the parasympathetic system never gets a chance to balance things out. High sympathetic drive can be linked to numerous chronic diseases both directly and indirectly.

However, by using breathing techniques to manipulate our ANS and help increase our parasympathetic drive, we can help manage our internal environment.

Exercise is a stressor. If you go straight from the gym, rush home to get changed, sit in traffic on the way to wherever you need to go, and then have a stressful day doing whatever you are doing, you are running on the edge. The body doesn't care where the stress comes from, it just keeps filling the cup until it's ready to tip over… speaking of cups, this is why so many people turn to alcohol in the evening. "It's just been such a big day!"

By having our members take two minutes at the end of their session to stop and slow their breathing down, we are trying to get them to leave the room in a relaxed state rather than bouncing from one stress to another.

It may only be for a couple of minutes, but it's at least a reminder of its importance and an easy task they can perform anywhere.

SECTION 4: RESOURCES

APPLYING THE HEALTH BELIEFS MODEL

This simple exercise will help you apply the **Health Belief Model** to a health behaviour you want to improve.

Step 1: Choose a Health Goal

Pick something specific, like:

- Walking more
- Eating healthier
- Strength training twice a week.

Step 2: Answer these key questions

1) **Perceived threat** – What happens if I don't change?
   Example: If I don't exercise, I might lose strength and balance as I age.

2) **Perceived benefits** – How will this help me?
   Example: Walking daily will keep me mobile and independent.

3) **Perceived barriers** – What could stop me?
   Example: I feel too tired, or I don't know where to start.

4) **Cues to action** – What can remind me to act?
   Example: Setting a daily reminder, joining a class, or having a walking buddy.

5) **Self-efficacy** – How confident am I that I can do this? What will help me succeed?
   Example: I'll start small, like a 10-minute walk, and build up.

Step 3: Make a small commitment

Write down one simple action you can take **today** to move toward your goal.

Example: I will take a 10-minute walk after breakfast.

By doing this, you're making behaviour change **practical, achievable, and personal.**

SETTING SMART GOALS

This activity is designed to help you set clear, realistic, and achievable exercise goals using the SMART (Specific, Measurable, Achievable, Relevant, Time-bound) framework — a scientifically backed method for behaviour change.

Step 1: Reflect on your current activity and readiness for change

Before setting goals, answer the following:

On average, how many days per week do you engage in physical activity?

☐ 0 days

☐ 1 – 2 days

☐ 3 – 4 days

☐ 5+ days

How much time do you spend being active per session?

☐ Less than 10 minutes

☐ 10 – 30 minutes

☐ 30 – 60 minutes

☐ More than 60 minutes

What types of activities do you currently do?
(Check all that apply)

☐ Walking

☐ Strength training

☐ Balance exercises (e.g., Tai Chi)

☐ Stretching/flexibility

☐ Recreational sports (e.g., tennis, golf)

☐ Other: __________

What barriers have prevented you from exercising more?
(Check all that apply)

☐ Lack of motivation

☐ Fear of injury/falling

☐ Lack of time

☐ Pain or discomfort

☐ Lack of support or guidance

☐ Other: __________

Step 2: Create a SMART Goal

Use the template below to create an exercise goal that suits your needs:

- **Specific** – What activity will you do?
- **Measurable** – How often? For how long?
- **Achievable** – Can you realistically meet this goal?
- **Relevant** – Does this align with your needs/interests?
- **Time-bound** – By when will you achieve this goal?

Example goal for a beginner:

"I will walk for 20 minutes, 3 times per week for the next month to improve my fitness and mobility."

Example goal for strength training:

"I will do a 15-minute resistance training session twice a week for the next 6 weeks to maintain my muscle strength and prevent falls."

Example goal for social engagement:

"I will join a group exercise class once a week for the next 8 weeks to stay active and build social connections."

Step 3: Plan for success

Identify support: Will you ask a friend or family member to join you?
Overcome barriers: How will you handle challenges (e.g. bad weather, low motivation)?
Track progress: Use a simple calendar or journal to check off completed sessions.
Adjust as needed: If your goal feels too easy or too hard, modify it for long-term success.

Step 4: Evaluate and celebrate progress

At the end of your set timeframe (e.g. 4, 6, or 8 weeks), reflect:

- Did you meet your goal? Why or why not?
- How do you feel physically and mentally?
- What will your next goal be?

HABIT CREATION TOOL

30-Day Habit Tracker

Use this visual tool to track your progress and build momentum.

Habit: ____

Week	Mon	Tue	Wed	Thu	Fri	Sat	Sun
Week 1							
Week 2							
Week 3							
Week 4							
Week 5							

CHAPTER 17

ONWARD & UPWARD

At the time of writing this book, I am reading a book called 'The Future Is Faster Than You Think', by Peter Diamandis and Steven Kotler. Among other incredible, technology-driven societal changes that they see coming our way, is the impact that technology, AI in particular, will have on health and disease management.

One of the greatest impacts of exercise, and its strongest selling point, is its ability to positively affect multiple systems at once. This is why there has never been a pill that has come close to mimicking it. However, based on what I'm reading, a 'return to youth' pill may not be such a fantasy after all. In the next ten or twenty years, we are going to see some monumental changes in pharmacological disease management. Let's hope that greed, money, and power don't get in the way of what could be lifesaving treatments for millions of people around the world.

> *"Never let the future disturb you. You will meet it, if you have to, with the same weapons of reason which today arm you against the present." – Marcus Aurelius*

One of the things that technology will not be able to replace is our need for human connection. Based on the increased rates of depression and anxiety we've seen attributed to social media use in teenagers, I'd hazard a guess that things might get worse.

As we've discussed, social interaction and maintaining positive social relationships can influence our quality of life in so many ways. To be able to now quantify this with the impact these things have on health markers such as stress, blood pressure, and all-cause mortality adds further weight to the argument.

The combination of exercise and social interaction is a powerful weapon in your longevity and health armoury. Social accountability, health behaviour change adherence, consistent exercise habits, positive relationship building, goal achievement, building physical confidence, improved ability to perform activities of daily living, and overall greater quality of life are just some of the benefits that can be obtained.

I am so grateful to be able to do what I do and am blessed to be able to witness people's lives and their health change before my very eyes. Thank you to those members who shared their stories with us. My hope is that you saw some of yourself or someone you know reflected in those stories.

It is never too late to start moving, and never too late to make new friends, or better yet, befriend someone new.

I've not uncovered anything new here. I'm simply sharing my knowledge, and our experience with Community Moves, to help add further support to the tide of literature and media encouraging people to move more and live healthier, happier lives.

There may be some amazing technological advancements coming our way soon that could potentially fix all of our modern lifestyle-related ailments. I guess it's a matter of how long you're willing to wait and what kind of condition you want to be in when they arrive.

There is no guarantee that the technology will arrive or that it will be as effective as hoped. There is, however, a mountain of conclusive evidence of the benefits of exercise and social interaction at any age.

Don't wait for tomorrow — get strong and social today.

REFERENCE LIST

[1] Australian Bureau of Statistics. (2025, September 26). *Life expectancy* (ABS Measuring What Matters). Retrieved from https://www.abs.gov.au/statistics/measuring-what-matters/measuring-what-matters-themes-and-indicators/healthy/life-expectancy

[2] NHMRC – Environment Scan. (2023, November). Health and nutrition of older Australians – Environment scan (Attachment A). Canberra: Commonwealth of Australia.

[3] Saltin, B., Blomqvist, G., Mitchell, J.H., Johnson, R.L. Jr., Wildenthal, K., & Chapman, C.B. (1968). *Response to exercise after bed rest and after training. Circulation*, 38(5 Suppl), VII1–VII78.

[4] McGuire, D.K., Levine, B.D., Williamson, J.W., et al. (2001). A 30-year follow-up of the Dallas Bed Rest and Training Study: II. Effect of age on cardiovascular adaptation to exercise training. *Circulation*, 104(12), 1358–1366.

[5] Pontzer, H., Raichlen, D. A., Wood, B. M., Mabulla, A. Z. P., Racette, S. B., Marlowe, F. W., … Zderic, T. W. (2018). Energy expenditure and activity among Hadza hunter-gatherers. *American Journal of Human Biology, 30*(2), e23142.

[6] HCF Health. (2024, August). *5 ways to reach your daily step goal.* https://www.hcf.com.au/health-agenda/body-mind/physical-health/ways-to-reach-your-daily-step-goal

[7] Australian Bureau of Statistics. (2023, December 15). *Physical activity, 2022* (Catalogue No. 4364.0).

[8] Australian Bureau of Statistics. (2023, December 15). *Health conditions prevalence, 2022* (Release). https://www.abs.gov.au/statistics/health/health-conditions-and-risks/health-conditions-prevalence/latest-release

[9] Lundberg, J. O., Settergren, G., Gelinder, S., Lundberg, J. M., Alving, K., & Weitzberg, E. (1996). Inhalation of nasally derived nitric oxide modulates pulmonary function in humans. *Acta Physiologica Scandinavica, 158*(4), 343-347.

[10] DeFronzo, R. A., Jacot, E., Jequier, E., Maeder, E., Wahren, J., & Felber, J. P. (1981). The effect of insulin on the disposal of intravenous glucose. *Diabetes, 30*(12), 1000–1007.

[11] Schnyder, S., & Handschin, C. (2015). Skeletal muscle as an endocrine organ: PGC-1α, myokines and… *Molecular Metabolism*, 4(4), 393-406.

[12] Rasmussen, P., Brassard, P., Adser, H., Pedersen, M. V., Leick, L., Hart, E., Secher, N. H., Pedersen, B. K., & Pilegaard, H. (2009). Evidence for a release of brain-derived neurotrophic factor from the brain during exercise. *Experimental Physiology, 94*(10), 1062–1069.

[13] Mitchell, W. K., Williams, J., Atherton, P., Larvin, M., Lund, J., & Narici, M. (2012). Sarcopenia, dynapenia, and the impact of advancing age on human skeletal muscle size and strength. *Age, 34*(2), 363–383.

[14] Moreland, J. D., Richardson, J. A., Goldsmith, C. H., & Clase, C. M. (2004). Muscle weakness and falls in older adults: A systematic review and meta-analysis. *Journal of the American Geriatrics Society, 52*(7), 1121–1129.

[15] Morris, J. N., Heady, J. A., Raffle, P. A. B., Roberts, C. G., & Parks, J. W. (1953). Coronary heart disease and physical activity of work. *The Lancet, 262*(6795), 1053–1057.

[16] Kodama, S., Saito, K., Tanaka, S., Maki, M., Yachi, Y., Asumi, M., … Sone, H. (2009). Cardiorespiratory fitness as a quantitative predictor of all-cause mortality and cardiovascular events in healthy men and women: A meta-analysis. JAMA, 301(19), 2024–2035.

[17] Sallis, R., Young, D. R., Tartof, S. Y., Sallis, J. F., Sall, J., Li, Q., Smith, G. N., & Cohen, D. A. (2021). Physical inactivity is associated with a higher risk for severe COVID-19 outcomes: A study in 48,440 adult patients. *British Journal of Sports Medicine, 55*(19), 1099–1105.

[18] Hightower, C. E., Benson, K. R., Chair, D., & Adesanya, A. O. (2020). Perioperative cardiovascular evaluation and management of patients undergoing noncardiac surgery. *Medical Clinics of North America, 104*(4), 663–677.

[19] Smith, R. L., Soeters, M. R., Wüst, R. C. I., & Houtkooper, R. H. (2018). Metabolic flexibility as an adaptation to energy resources and requirements in health and disease. Endocrine Reviews, 39(4), 489–517.

[20] Balance and walking speed predict subsequent 8-year mortality by Blain et al. (2010) — shows that poor balance and mobility significantly predicted 8-year mortality in older adults.

[21] Australian Institute of Health and Welfare. (2022). Falls in older Australians 2019–20: Hospitalisations and deaths among people aged 65 and over. Canberra: AIHW.

[22] Australian Orthopaedic Association National Joint Replacement Registry (AOANJRR). (2021). *Annual Report 2021 – Hip, Knee & Shoulder Arthroplasty.*

[23] Harris, I. A., Cuthbert, A., Lorimer, M., de Steiger, R., Lewis, P. L., Graves, S. E. (2019). How does mortality risk change over time after hip and knee arthroplasty? *Clinical Orthopaedics and Related Research, 477*(6), 1414-1421.

[24] Verdquin-David, M., et al. (2020). Effects of saccadic eye movements on balance control in older adults. *Experimental Brain Research, 238*(10), 2297–2306.

[25] Borde, R., Hortobágyi, T., & Granacher, U. (2015). Dose–response relationships of resistance training in healthy old adults: A systematic review and meta-analysis. *Sports Medicine, 45*, 1693–1720.

[26] Schiaffino, S., & Reggiani, C. (2011). Fiber types in mammalian skeletal muscles. *Physiological Reviews, 91*(4), 1447–1531.

[27] Lexell, J., Taylor, C. C., & Sjöström, M. (1988). What is the cause of the ageing atrophy? Total number, size and proportion of different fiber types studied in whole vastus lateralis muscle from 15- to 83-year-old men. *Journal of the Neurological Sciences, 84*(2–3), 275–294.

[28] Schoenfeld, B. J., Pope, Z. K., Benik, F. M., Hester, G. M., Sellers, J., Nooner, J. L., Schnaiter, J. A., Bond-Williams, K. E., Carter, A. S., Ross, C. L., Just, B. L., Henselmans, M., & Krieger, J. W. (2016). Longer inter-set rest periods enhance muscle strength and hypertrophy in resistance-trained men. *Journal of Strength and Conditioning Research, 30*(7), 1805–1812.

[29] Carroll, T. J., Selvanayagam, V. S., Riek, S., & Semmler, J. G. (2011). Neural adaptations to strength training: Moving beyond transcranial magnetic stimulation and reflex studies. *Acta Physiologica, 202*(2), 119–140.

[30] Kortebein, P., Symons, T. B., Ferrando, A., Paddon-Jones, D., Ronsen, O., Protas, E., Conger, S., Lombeida, J., Wolfe, R., & Evans, W. J. (2008). *Functional impact of 10 days of bed rest in healthy older adults.* Journals of Gerontology – Series A: Biological Sciences and Medical Sciences, 63(10), 1076-1081.

[31] Bauer, J., Biolo, G., Cederholm, T., Cesari, M., Cruz-Jentoft, A., Morley, J. E., Phillips, S., Sieber, C., Stehle, P., Teta, D., Visvanathan, R., & Volpi, E. (2013).Evidence-based recommendations for optimal dietary protein intake in older people. *Journal of the American Medical Directors Association, 14*(8), 542–559.

[32] Holt-Lunstad, J., Smith, T. B., Baker, M., Harris, T., & Stephenson, D. (2015). Loneliness and social isolation as risk factors for mortality: A meta-analytic review. *Perspectives on Psychological Science, 10*(2), 227–237.

[33] AIFS. (2020). Social isolation and loneliness: Insights from Australian research. https://aifs.gov.au/resources/research-snapshot/social-isolation-factors-dynamics-and-effects-isolation-older-people

[34] Social Relationships and Mortality Risk: A Meta-analytic Review (Holt-Lunstad, Smith & Layton, 2010) — published in PLOS Medicine

[35] Yang, Y. C., Boen, C., Gerken, K., Li, T., Schorpp, K., & Harris, K. M. (2016). Social relationships and physiological determinants of longevity across the human life span. *Proceedings of the National Academy of Sciences, 113*(3), 578–583.

[36] Prochaska, J. O., & Velicer, W. F. (1997). The transtheoretical model of health behavior change. *American Journal of Health Promotion, 12*(1), 38–48.

[37] Rosenstock, I. M. (1974). Historical origins of the Health Belief Model. *Health Education Monographs, 2*(4), 328–335.

[38] Bronfenbrenner, U. (1977). Toward an experimental ecology of human development. *American Psychologist, 32*(7), 513–531.

[39] Kelley, R. E., & Conner, D. R. (1979). Emotional stages of change. Positively Managing Organizational Transitions.

www.ingramcontent.com/pod-product-compliance
Lightning Source LLC
LaVergne TN
LVHW020045110826
845155LV00029B/639

* 9 7 8 1 9 2 3 6 5 0 2 0 6 *